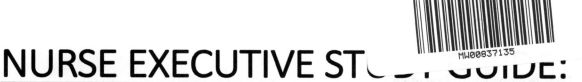

# NURSE EXECUTIVE STUDY GUIDE:

## INTRODUCTION:

Dear Aspiring Nurse Executive,

Everyone has a dream, a guiding light that beckons them toward a future where they not only succeed but thrive. Your dream, of taking on the mantle of Nurse Executive, is a noble and challenging aspiration, and you are not alone on this journey.

Every great endeavor begins with a spark, an inner calling. Perhaps yours is a deep-seated desire to shape the world of healthcare, or maybe it's the passion to lead and inspire a generation of nurses. Yet, with dreams come uncertainties, doubts, and the inevitable challenges that may sometimes seem insurmountable. It's natural to question whether you've taken the right path or if you have what it takes to realize your ambition.

This book isn't just a testament to the knowledge you need to embark on your journey; it's a companion. In moments of doubt, it provides understanding; in times of challenge, it offers solace. At the crossroads of uncertainty, it stands to validate your feelings, reassuring you that every Nurse Executive, before becoming a beacon of leadership, grappled with the same thoughts.

As you delve into these pages, remember that the path to greatness is seldom straightforward. There will be hurdles and setbacks, but also moments of clarity, inspiration, and triumph. Each page of this guide is crafted to fuel your aspirations, instilling in you the belief that your dream is not just attainable but absolutely worth every ounce of effort.

Your passion and dedication are the wind beneath the wings of your dream. This guide is but a tool, a stepping stone in your larger voyage. Embrace the journey, cherish the learning, and always remember - your aspirations, combined with your determination and the right resources, are a force to be reckoned with.

Together, let's journey towards your dream, for the world of healthcare awaits your leadership, vision, and transformative touch.

### Introduction to the Nurse Executive Role
The Nurse Executive Role, as recognized within the nursing community, is a pivotal position that combines the multifaceted realms of clinical expertise, leadership prowess, and administrative acumen. It's a role poised at the intersection of patient care, team management, and strategic healthcare visions.
### Core Competencies:
1. **Strategic Vision**: Nurse executives craft and implement visionary strategies that resonate with the larger goals of the healthcare institution. They are not just reactive

but proactive in anticipating the future of healthcare and setting the direction accordingly.

2. **Clinical Practice Knowledge**: While they might not be directly involved in bedside care, their clinical judgment remains impeccable. Their decisions are informed by clinical best practices, ensuring patient safety and optimum care standards.

3. **Financial Acumen**: From budgeting to understanding the economic landscape of healthcare, nurse executives juggle numbers with precision. This is crucial, as decisions often need to balance clinical excellence with economic viability.

4. **Human Resource Management**: Managing a diverse nursing team requires a nuanced understanding of human behavior, team dynamics, conflict resolution, and motivational strategies. Ensuring that the nursing staff is equipped, empowered, and engaged is a continuous task.

5. **Regulatory and Compliance Knowledge**: U.S. healthcare is governed by myriad regulations, from federal mandates like the Health Insurance Portability and Accountability Act (HIPAA) to state-specific nursing guidelines. Nurse executives ensure adherence, which is pivotal not just for legal compliance but also for maintaining the institution's reputation.

**Real-world Application**: Consider the introduction of a new medical technology in a hospital. While the clinical staff might be excited about its potential, the nurse executive plays a crucial role in training, budget considerations, regulatory compliance, and measuring its impact on patient care outcomes. Their perspective is holistic, ensuring that every new venture aligns with the institution's mission and values.

**Evolving Landscape**: With healthcare's rapid evolution, particularly in the realms of digital health and telemedicine, the role of the nurse executive has expanded. They are often at the forefront of integrating these technologies, ensuring that while innovation thrives, patient care remains uncompromised.

In essence, the Nurse Executive stands as a beacon, guiding and governing the nursing realm within the complex machinery of modern healthcare. Their decisions, insights, and leadership mold the present and future of patient care, staff well-being, and the healthcare institution's overarching trajectory.

**Exam Pointer**: When preparing for the ANCC Nurse Executive exam, it's essential to grasp not just the theoretical aspects of the role but also the real-world challenges and solutions that nurse executives encounter. Delving into case studies, understanding healthcare economics, and keeping abreast of recent regulatory changes will serve you well in mastering the content and excelling in the examination.

### Overview of the ANCC Nurse Executive Exam

The ANCC Nurse Executive exam stands as a rigorous assessment, meticulously designed to evaluate the knowledge and skills of nursing leaders. Its structure and content mirror the multifaceted role of Nurse Executives in today's ever-evolving healthcare landscape.

1. **Exam Composition**: The test consists of 175 questions. However, only 150 of these are scored, with the remaining 25 serving as potential questions for future exams. These

non-scored questions are scattered throughout the exam, and test-takers won't be able to distinguish them from scored ones.

2. **Content Areas**:
   - **Structural and Organizational Elements** (22%): Encompasses staffing, workload considerations, and the principles governing effective leadership and governance.
   - **Leadership and Professional Practice** (28%): Centers on leadership theories, conflict resolution, communication, and ethics.
   - **Communication and Relationship Management** (20%): Delves into communication strategies, interdisciplinary collaboration, and patient advocacy.
   - **Knowledge of the Healthcare Environment** (18%): Addresses current healthcare trends, regulations, and the broader healthcare system.
   - **Business Skills** (12%): Evaluates understanding of financial management, strategic planning, and risk management.

3. **Test Duration**: Candidates have a generous 3.5 hours to complete the exam, allowing ample time for thoughtful consideration of each question.

4. **Scoring Mechanism**: The test uses a criterion-referenced method. This means scores are not curved. The raw score (number of correctly answered questions) is transformed into a scaled score. A score of 350 out of 500 is the minimum passing score.

5. **Exam Delivery**: The exam is computer-based and is offered at designated testing centers worldwide.

6. **Preparation Tips**:
   - **Focus on Practical Knowledge**: Real-world scenarios often grace the pages of the exam, testing not just theoretical knowledge but its application.
   - **Stay Updated**: With healthcare in constant flux, being aware of the latest trends, regulations, and methodologies is paramount.

**Technical Insight**: Did you know that the Nurse Executive exam is updated periodically to reflect the most recent changes in the field? A panel of experts meticulously reviews the content to ensure its relevance and accuracy.

Approaching this exam, it's not just about memorizing facts but assimilating knowledge and applying it contextually. Your success will be a testament to your mastery, positioning you as a leader ready to shape the future of healthcare.

**Eligibility and Application Process for the ANCC Nurse Executive Exam**
**Eligibility Criteria**:
1. **Current Active RN License**: This is paramount. You must possess an active RN license (or equivalent from another country) to apply.
2. **Educational Requirements**:
   - **Option A**: Baccalaureate or higher degree in nursing and two years full-time equivalent practice as a registered nurse in an administrative position within the

last five years. Also, you must have completed 30 hours of continuing education in nursing administration within the last three years.
- **Option B**: Non-nursing baccalaureate degree, a master's degree in nursing, two years full-time equivalent practice as an RN in an administrative position within the last five years, and 30 hours of continuing education in nursing administration within the last three years.

3. **Professional Experience**: Depending on the educational background, the required work experience varies. The essence is hands-on administrative experience, ensuring the candidate is well-versed with real-world challenges and solutions.

**Application Process:**
1. **Online Application**: Begin by visiting the ANCC website. The application process is predominantly online, streamlined for user convenience.
2. **Supporting Documents**: It's vital to have scanned copies of required documents, especially your RN license, educational certificates, and proof of work experience.
3. **Fees**: Application fees vary based on your membership status with the American Nurses Association (ANA) and other affiliated organizations. Regular applicants might face a higher fee compared to ANA members.
4. **Verification Process**: After submission, the ANCC will review the application. This verification process checks the accuracy of submitted details, ensuring only eligible candidates proceed.
5. **Scheduling the Exam**: Once approved, you will receive a notification with instructions to schedule your examination through a designated testing service.
6. **Retesting**: If, for any reason, a candidate does not pass the exam on the first attempt, there's a provision to retake it. However, retesting requires a waiting period and may involve additional fees.

By understanding these eligibility and application nuances, aspiring Nurse Executives can confidently navigate the path to certification, ensuring they're adequately prepared to lead and innovate in the nursing realm.

**Exam Format and Duration for the ANCC Nurse Executive Exam**
**Format:**
1. **Type of Questions**: The exam predominantly consists of multiple-choice questions, requiring candidates to select the best answer from the provided options.
2. **Number of Questions**: There are typically 175 questions on the test, but only 150 of these are scored. The remaining 25 are pretest questions being evaluated for future exams and don't count towards your final score.
3. **Content Breakdown**: Questions are structured around key domain areas essential for nurse executives. These domains can include leadership, structural and organizational skills, communication, knowledge management, professionalism, and business skills.

**Duration:** The total exam time is approximately 3.5 hours. This time encompasses test-taking, any breaks, and tutorial instructions.

**Test-Taking Strategies and Tips**:
1. **Understand the Blueprint**: Familiarize yourself with the content outline of the exam available on the ANCC website. Knowing what to expect gives you a strategic advantage.
2. **Practice with Mock Tests**: Sample questions and mock tests not only help you get accustomed to the format but also help in time management. You'll be able to gauge areas that need more focus.
3. **Read Questions Carefully**: Given the multiple-choice format, subtle differences in wording can lead to dramatically different interpretations.
4. **Time Management**: With 3.5 hours and 175 questions, you have roughly 1.2 minutes per question. Regularly checking the clock ensures you don't spend too much time on a single question.
5. **Educated Guessing**: If you don't know an answer, don't leave the question blank. Eliminate the choices that you know are incorrect and make an educated guess. There's no penalty for wrong answers.
6. **Stay Calm and Centered**: Anxiety can cloud judgment. Deep breathing, taking short breaks if needed, and maintaining a positive mindset can make a significant difference.
7. **Plan Ahead**: Ensure you're familiar with the test location. Arrive early, bringing along any required identification.
8. **Real-world Relevance**: When tackling scenario-based questions, try relating them to real-world situations or experiences you've encountered or heard about. This can often offer clarity on the best choices.
9. **Post-Question Reflection**: After the exam, refrain from dwelling on questions that you found challenging. Every candidate has unique strengths and areas for improvement. Focus on the learning journey and the steps ahead.

By thoroughly preparing and employing these strategies, candidates can approach the ANCC Nurse Executive Exam with confidence and poise, enhancing their chances of success.

# **Structural and Organizational Environment:**

### Introduction to Governance in Healthcare Organizations
Governance, in the context of healthcare organizations, refers to the system of practices, processes, and policies that direct and control an institution. It encompasses the way duties and responsibilities are assigned among different roles, how decisions are made, and the mechanisms to align them with the facility's mission, vision, and strategy.

Foundational Concepts of Governance:
1. **Accountability**: The obligation of individuals or groups to report their activities, accept responsibility for them, and disclose the results transparently.
2. **Stewardship**: Refers to the leadership's commitment to ethical and responsible decision-making, ensuring the welfare of all stakeholders.
3. **Transparency**: Decision-making processes are open and clear, enabling stakeholders to have an understanding of the proceedings.

4. **Inclusiveness**: Ensuring diverse perspectives are considered, which often requires the inclusion of community members, medical staff, and other stakeholders in decisions.

**Impact on Daily Operations:**
1. **Policy Implementation**: Governance lays down policies that every department in a healthcare facility must adhere to. This can include everything from patient care protocols to employee conduct.
2. **Resource Allocation**: Governance decisions directly impact how resources, including funding and manpower, are allocated across the facility.
3. **Risk Management**: Governance frameworks identify and mitigate risks, ensuring patient safety and organizational stability.
4. **Quality Assurance**: Governance systems ensure that the healthcare facility meets or exceeds established standards, leading to continuous improvement in patient care.

**Historical Evolution of Governance in Healthcare:**
- **Early Models (Pre-20th Century)**: Governance was typically a solo endeavor where individual physicians or groups operated their practices. Hospitals were often charity-based and overseen by religious or philanthropic groups.
- **Mid 20th Century**: With the rise of healthcare as a system, there was an increased need for organized, formal governance structures. Hospitals started to have boards, often comprised of prominent local figures, without significant healthcare expertise.
- **Late 20th Century**: The increasing complexity of healthcare, both clinically and economically, led to a more professional approach to governance. Hospitals merged, leading to larger systems requiring formalized structures. There was an emphasis on including medical professionals in the decision-making processes.
- **21st Century**: Today, governance in healthcare is seen as a partnership between administrative professionals and medical staff. With the rise of patient-centered care, there's a growing emphasis on including patient perspectives in governance. There's also a strong focus on transparency, ethics, and social responsibility, given the heightened public scrutiny.

In the current landscape, the effective governance of healthcare organizations isn't merely a regulatory requirement but a keystone for achieving excellence in patient care, employee satisfaction, and community trust. Whether it's a major hospital in a metropolitan area or a rural clinic, the principles of governance remain crucial to ensuring that every patient receives the best care possible.

**Roles and Responsibilities in Healthcare Governance**
1. **Board of Directors/Trustees:**
    - **Responsibilities**: Strategic oversight, financial stewardship, policy approval, executive hiring and evaluation, risk management, and ensuring quality care.
    - They usually have sub-committees like finance, audit, and quality assurance.
2. **Chief Executive Officer (CEO):**

- **Responsibilities**: Day-to-day management, executing the board's strategies, leading senior management, and being the primary liaison between the board and the staff.
3. **Chief Medical Officer (CMO)**:
   - **Responsibilities**: Oversee clinical practices, advocate for patient safety and care quality, liaise between medical staff and executive management, and influence policy decisions related to clinical practices.
4. **Chief Nursing Officer (CNO)**:
   - **Responsibilities**: Oversee nursing practices, ensure patient care quality, advocate for nursing staff's professional development and well-being, and contribute to policy decisions related to nursing.
5. **Other C-suite executives (e.g., CFO, CIO)**:
   - **Responsibilities**: Oversee specific departments like finance or IT, collaborate with other executives to ensure alignment of departmental goals with organizational goals.
6. **Medical Staff Leadership**:
   - **Responsibilities**: Represent the interests and concerns of the medical staff, liaise with management, contribute to policy decisions, and ensure the highest standards of clinical care.

**Collaboration for Organizational Effectiveness**:

Roles within healthcare governance don't operate in isolation. For a healthcare organization to function optimally:

- The **Board** sets strategic directions and policies.
- The **CEO** operationalizes these strategies, often with input and collaboration from the CMO, CNO, and other C-suite executives.
- The **CMO** and **CNO** ensure that these strategies align with the best clinical practices, ensuring patient safety and care quality.
- **Medical Staff Leadership** gives voice to the clinicians' perspectives, ensuring that the strategies and policies set are practical, realistic, and prioritize patient care.

**Importance of Clear Role Delineation**:

1. **Prevents Overlaps**: Ensures that tasks aren't duplicated, leading to efficient use of resources.
2. **Minimizes Gaps**: Ensures that no task is overlooked.
3. **Enhances Accountability**: When roles are clear, it's evident who is responsible for what. This clarity drives performance and ensures that individuals or teams are accountable for their areas.
4. **Streamlines Decision-making**: In situations demanding quick decisions, clearly defined roles mean that the right person can make the decision without delays.
5. **Promotes Professional Growth**: When staff understand their roles and the scope of their responsibilities, they can focus on their professional development in their specific areas.

Clear delineation of roles and responsibilities is not just a governance best practice. In healthcare, where lives are often at stake, it becomes a critical component for ensuring efficient, effective, and patient-centered care.

**Governance Structures in Healthcare Organizations**

Governance in healthcare is typically a multi-layered structure designed to ensure patient safety, quality of care, financial stability, and adherence to regulations. The common structures are:

1. **Board of Directors/Trustees**: Typically the highest decision-making body, the Board has ultimate responsibility for the organization's strategic direction, fiscal integrity, and performance outcomes. They approve budgets, oversee the CEO, and ensure legal and ethical compliance.
2. **Executive Management (C-suite)**: Led by the CEO, this group includes the Chief Medical Officer (CMO), Chief Nursing Officer (CNO), Chief Financial Officer (CFO), and other high-level managers. They're responsible for day-to-day operations and executing the Board's strategies.
3. **Medical Staff Governance**: This includes Medical Executive Committees and department chairs, representing physicians and clinical staff. They oversee credentialing, peer reviews, and quality improvement initiatives specific to clinical care.
4. **Committees**: There can be numerous committees, each dedicated to a specific area, like quality assurance, ethics, finance, audit, or credentials. They ensure specialized oversight and guide policy-making.

**Mechanisms Supporting Governance Structures**:

1. **Bylaws**: Each governance structure has its bylaws outlining its composition, authority, duties, and operations. Bylaws ensure consistency and clarity in function.
2. **Policies and Procedures**: These are detailed documents that provide guidelines for decision-making and actions within various governance structures.
3. **Performance Metrics and Dashboards**: These tools help in monitoring and assessing the performance of various departments, guiding decisions, and ensuring accountability.
4. **Regular Meetings**: Scheduled meetings ensure continual communication and coordination among the different governance bodies.
5. **Education and Training**: Regular updates on regulatory changes, best practices, and performance outcomes keep members informed and effective.
6. **Feedback Mechanisms**: Systems for obtaining feedback from patients, staff, and other stakeholders help in decision-making and improving service delivery.

**Adapting to Changes in the Healthcare Environment**:

The healthcare landscape is continually evolving due to technological advances, regulatory changes, patient expectations, and other external factors. Governance structures must adapt in response.

1. **Strategic Planning Sessions**: These sessions help in reassessing the organization's direction based on current realities. They may result in a change in focus, the introduction of new services, or even discontinuation of certain practices.

2. **Integration of Technology**: New health information systems or telehealth platforms may necessitate changes in how care is delivered, monitored, and evaluated.
3. **Regulatory Compliance**: Changes in healthcare laws or standards may require governance structures to review and modify policies, procedures, and practices.
4. **Collaborative Partnerships**: As healthcare becomes more integrated, governance might need to account for collaborations or mergers with other healthcare entities.
5. **Continuous Education**: Governance members must be updated on the latest trends, challenges, and opportunities in healthcare to make informed decisions.

Understanding governance structures and mechanisms is essential for nurse executives. They must navigate these structures effectively, ensuring that nursing's voice is heard, and that decisions align with best practices and optimal patient outcomes.

**Defining Organizational Culture in Healthcare**

Organizational culture in healthcare refers to the shared values, beliefs, behaviors, customs, and attitudes that characterize an institution and guide its practices. It's the "way things are done here" – an intangible force that shapes behaviors, decision-making, and overall dynamics within a healthcare environment. It includes how staff communicate, how risks are managed, how successes are celebrated, and even how failures are addressed.

**Influence of Organizational Culture on Decision-making**

1. **Values and Beliefs**: At its core, an organization's shared values and beliefs influence the choices made. For instance, if a hospital's culture strongly values patient-centered care, decisions regarding resource allocation, hiring, or treatment protocols will prioritize patient needs and preferences.
2. **Risk Tolerance**: Organizations with a risk-averse culture might hesitate to adopt new technologies or therapies until they're well-established. Conversely, a culture open to innovation may be more willing to explore cutting-edge treatments or methodologies.
3. **Communication Patterns**: In cultures that encourage open communication, decision-making tends to be more collaborative. Staff at all levels feel empowered to voice opinions and share insights. In contrast, hierarchical cultures might see decisions made predominantly by top-level management without much input from frontline staff.
4. **Reward Systems**: If the culture emphasizes certain outcomes (e.g., patient satisfaction scores), decision-making will tilt towards achieving those outcomes, sometimes even at the cost of other equally important factors.

**Relationship Between Governance and Organizational Culture:**

1. **Setting the Tone**: Governance bodies, especially the Board and executive management, play a crucial role in defining an organization's culture. Their values, behaviors, and decisions cascade down, influencing all levels of the organization.
2. **Policy and Procedures**: Governance determines the policies and procedures of an institution. These documents are both a reflection of the existing culture and a tool to shape it. For example, a policy that mandates regular team huddles or feedback sessions indicates a culture that values communication and collaboration.

3. **Accountability**: Governance structures hold various departments and individuals accountable. This accountability can either foster a culture of blame or a culture of continuous improvement, depending on how failures or shortcomings are addressed.
4. **Resource Allocation**: The way governance allocates resources – be it for training, new technologies, or patient care initiatives – showcases what the organization values, thereby reinforcing certain cultural attributes.
5. **Response to External Changes**: How governance reacts to external pressures, whether they're regulatory changes or public health crises, also shapes culture. For example, a proactive response to a pandemic situation, prioritizing staff safety and patient care, strengthens a culture of agility and care.

In essence, governance and organizational culture are deeply interwoven. Governance not only reflects the existing culture but also holds the power to shape and evolve it to better meet the needs of patients, staff, and other stakeholders.

**Strategies Employed by Governance Bodies to Promote Safety and Excellence:**
1. **Implementation of Evidence-Based Protocols**: Governance bodies often adopt and enforce evidence-based protocols and best practices, ensuring that the most current and effective methods are in use.
2. **Regular Audits and Evaluations**: By routinely auditing clinical practices and outcomes, governance can identify areas of concern and work towards rectification.
3. **Promotion of Open Communication**: Encouraging transparent reporting of errors or near misses without fear of retribution can lead to a proactive approach in addressing potential risks.
4. **Investment in Training and Development**: Ensuring that staff are well-trained not only in their clinical roles but also in safety protocols and new technologies is crucial.
5. **Patient Engagement**: Governance can employ strategies to include patients' perspectives, such as patient satisfaction surveys and feedback mechanisms, to improve overall care quality.

**Ensuring Compliance with Safety Regulations and Standards:**
1. **Establishment of Dedicated Committees**: Governance bodies often establish committees focused on quality and safety. These committees regularly review policies, processes, and outcomes to ensure alignment with safety standards.
2. **Regular Reporting**: Mandated periodic reporting on safety metrics, adverse events, and other quality indicators helps in keeping track of the institution's performance against established benchmarks.
3. **Liaison with Regulatory Bodies**: Regular interactions and collaborations with regulatory entities, like the Joint Commission, can ensure the organization remains updated on the latest safety standards and regulations.
4. **Accreditation and Certification**: Many governance bodies pursue voluntary accreditations and certifications that require adherence to high safety and quality standards.

**Role of Governance in Fostering a Culture of Continuous Improvement:**

1. **Leadership Buy-In**: Governance plays a pivotal role in demonstrating commitment to continuous improvement. When leadership is visibly involved in and supportive of improvement initiatives, it sets the tone for the entire organization.
2. **Resource Allocation**: Governance ensures the allocation of necessary resources – time, personnel, and finances – for quality improvement projects.
3. **Performance Metrics**: The establishment of clear performance metrics allows organizations to track progress and areas in need of attention. Governance often reviews these metrics to ensure alignment with the organization's strategic goals.
4. **Recognition and Reward Systems**: Celebrating successes and acknowledging teams or individuals who excel in their efforts towards continuous improvement can drive motivation and commitment across the board.
5. **Feedback Loops**: Governance supports mechanisms that enable feedback from frontline staff, patients, and other stakeholders. This feedback is invaluable in understanding the ground realities and areas of potential enhancement.

Real-world example: A hospital might implement a "Safety Huddle" initiative, a short, stand-up meeting held at the start of each shift, where teams discuss potential safety concerns for the day. Such a practice, when endorsed by governance, can empower staff at all levels to be vigilant about safety and voice concerns freely, promoting a proactive approach to safety and excellence.

**Signs Indicating a Need for Change in Organizational Culture:**
1. **High Turnover Rates**: When staff leave frequently, it might point to dissatisfaction, burnout, or a disconnect with the organization's values and culture.
2. **Increased Patient Complaints**: A surge in patient grievances can be indicative of systemic issues or an eroding culture of care.
3. **Lack of Collaboration**: Siloed departments or teams, resistance to interdisciplinary collaboration, or frequent conflicts signal cultural issues.
4. **Decreased Employee Engagement**: Low participation in organizational events, training, or feedback mechanisms suggests a potential disconnect.
5. **Safety and Compliance Incidents**: Increased incidents of safety breaches or non-compliance with protocols hint at deeper cultural problems.

**Steps for Governance to Initiate Culture Change:**
1. **Acknowledge the Need**: The first step is recognizing and admitting that there's a need for cultural transformation.
2. **Engage External Experts**: Consider hiring consultants or experts in organizational development to assess the current state and recommend strategies.
3. **Gather Input**: Engage staff at all levels, from frontline workers to managers, through surveys, focus groups, or open forums to understand their perspectives.
4. **Set Clear Vision and Goals**: Articulate a clear vision for the desired culture. This vision should align with the organization's mission and values.
5. **Develop a Strategic Action Plan**: This should include specific actions, timelines, responsible parties, and measurable outcomes.

6. **Communication**: Keep the lines of communication open at all stages. Inform staff about why the change is necessary, what's expected, and how it will benefit everyone.
7. **Leadership Modeling**: Leaders should model the desired behaviors and values, setting a tone for the entire organization.
8. **Ongoing Training and Development**: Equip staff with the skills, knowledge, and tools they need to adapt to the new cultural norms.
9. **Monitor and Adjust**: Regularly evaluate the progress of cultural change initiatives and adjust strategies as necessary.

**Supporting Staff During Cultural Transition:**
1. **Open Dialogue**: Encourage staff to voice their concerns, fears, or suggestions. This can be facilitated through town-hall meetings, feedback sessions, or suggestion boxes.
2. **Provide Resources**: Offer workshops, counseling, or training sessions to help staff navigate the changes and understand the new expectations.
3. **Recognition and Reward**: Acknowledge and celebrate those who champion and exemplify the new cultural values.
4. **Create Transition Teams**: These teams, often made up of early adopters or culture champions, can support their peers through the transition, acting as mentors or guides.
5. **Stay Transparent**: Be open about the reasons for change, the benefits expected, and the challenges foreseen. This reduces uncertainty and fosters trust.

Real-world example: A renowned healthcare facility, after noticing declining patient satisfaction scores and high staff turnover, conducted a series of focus groups and discovered a disconnect between frontline staff and leadership. To address this, the governance body implemented a program where leaders would regularly spend time on the floor, engaging with staff and patients alike. This "back to the floor" initiative bridged communication gaps, provided leaders with firsthand insights, and gradually shifted the organizational culture towards greater collaboration and transparency.

**Key Principles Behind Organizational Design in Healthcare:**
1. **Alignment with Mission and Vision**: The design should facilitate the institution's overarching goals and vision. It's the roadmap to achieving strategic initiatives.
2. **Patient-Centeredness**: The primary focus remains on delivering high-quality patient care. The design should promote efficiency, safety, and positive patient outcomes.
3. **Flexibility**: Healthcare is an ever-evolving field. The design must be adaptable to new technologies, regulations, and patient needs.
4. **Interdisciplinary Collaboration**: An effective design promotes collaboration across different disciplines, ensuring comprehensive care.
5. **Clear Reporting Hierarchies**: There should be clarity on roles, responsibilities, and reporting lines to ensure accountability.
6. **Scalability**: As healthcare organizations grow and diversify, the design should allow for expansion or reconfiguration without significant disruptions.

**How Organizational Structure Supports the Institution's Mission and Vision:**

The organizational structure is the backbone that holds the institution's goals, values, and strategies. A well-designed structure:

- Facilitates communication across different departments, ensuring that the institution's objectives are consistently understood and pursued.
- Ensures resources – both human and material – are optimally utilized towards fulfilling the mission.
- Provides clarity in roles, ensuring every member understands their contribution towards the larger vision.

For instance, a healthcare institution with a mission to provide comprehensive care might adopt an interdisciplinary team-based structure, wherein professionals from different specialties collaborate closely on patient care.

**Interplay between Governance and Organizational Design:**

Governance and organizational design are tightly interwoven. Here's how:

1. **Direction Setting**: Governance bodies set the strategic direction, and the organizational design is the tool to operationalize it.
2. **Resource Allocation**: Governance decides on the allocation of resources. The design ensures these resources are used where they're most impactful.
3. **Performance Monitoring**: The governance body uses the structure to monitor performance, ensuring departments and teams align with institutional goals.
4. **Policy Implementation**: Policies formulated by governance are implemented through the organizational structure. For instance, a policy on patient safety would require clear communication lines and collaboration, aspects determined by the design.
5. **Feedback Loop**: The organizational design provides a feedback mechanism to governance. Challenges in the design can be escalated to governance for resolution.
6. **Change Management**: When governance decides on transformative changes, the organizational design must be re-evaluated and possibly restructured to accommodate these changes.

*Real-world example*: A large teaching hospital aiming to become a leader in research might undergo a governance-directed redesign. This could lead to the establishment of a research department, allocation of resources for labs, and collaboration mechanisms between researchers and clinicians. The design facilitates the hospital's vision, while governance ensures it stays on track.

**Types of Organizational Designs in Healthcare Institutions:**

1. **Functional Design**:
   - **Description**: Departments are organized based on the functions they perform, e.g., nursing, radiology, administration.
   - **Pros**: Clear hierarchies, specialized teams, efficient for large organizations.
   - **Cons**: Can lead to silos, might inhibit inter-departmental collaboration, potential for duplicated efforts.
2. **Divisional Design**:

- **Description**: Departments are organized based on products, services, or patient demographics, e.g., pediatrics, geriatrics, orthopedics.
- **Pros**: Focus on specific patient populations, facilitates specialized care, clearer accountability.
- **Cons**: Might lead to resource duplication across divisions, can limit knowledge sharing.

3. **Matrix Design**:
   - **Description**: Combines functional and divisional designs, where professionals report to both a function head and a product/service lead.
   - **Pros**: Promotes inter-departmental collaboration, flexible, draws on strengths of both functional and divisional designs.
   - **Cons**: Dual reporting can lead to confusion, potential for conflicts, requires robust communication mechanisms.

4. **Flat Design**:
   - **Description**: Fewer levels of hierarchy, teams have more autonomy.
   - **Pros**: Faster decision-making, promotes employee empowerment, flexible.
   - **Cons**: Can be challenging for very large organizations, potential for role ambiguity.

5. **Team-Based Design**:
   - **Description**: Organized around teams rather than functions or services. Teams are usually interdisciplinary.
   - **Pros**: Encourages collaboration, adaptable to changing patient needs, can foster innovation.
   - **Cons**: Might lack clear hierarchy, requires robust team management, potential for role overlap.

6. **Network Design**:
   - **Description**: Consists of individual organizations or units that operate independently but collaborate on specific functions or projects.
   - **Pros**: Highly flexible, allows for specialization, scalable.
   - **Cons**: Control can be challenging, relies heavily on trust and communication, potential for fragmented services.

**Choosing the Most Appropriate Design for an Organization:**

A governance body should consider the following when choosing an organizational design:

1. **Organization's Goals and Vision**: Align the design with the institution's mission. For instance, if interdisciplinary care is a goal, a team-based design might be apt.
2. **Size and Scale**: Larger institutions might benefit from a functional or divisional structure, while smaller, agile institutions might opt for flat or team-based designs.
3. **Complexity**: For institutions offering a diverse range of services, matrix or network designs can be effective.
4. **Environment and External Factors**: If the external environment is rapidly changing, flexible designs like matrix or team-based might be preferable.

5. **Internal Dynamics**: Consider the institution's culture. An organization that values autonomy might thrive in a flat or team-based design.
6. **Feedback from Stakeholders**: Engage clinicians, staff, and patients to understand their needs and preferences.

*Real-world example*: A community healthcare center focusing on holistic care might opt for a team-based design, where a patient is seen by a team comprising a general physician, a nutritionist, a physical therapist, and a mental health professional. This facilitates comprehensive care while promoting collaboration among professionals.

**Impacts on Patient Care Quality:**
1. **Governance Oversight**: Governance ensures that clinical guidelines, safety protocols, and care standards are not just set but diligently followed. A governance body that emphasizes evidence-based practices typically ensures higher quality care.
2. **Resource Allocation**: Governance decisions on resource allocation—like hiring specialized staff or investing in cutting-edge equipment—can directly boost patient care quality. For instance, governance's decision to invest in telehealth can greatly benefit patients in remote areas.
3. **Accountability Mechanisms**: Effective governance structures establish accountability mechanisms, ensuring that deviations from care standards are promptly addressed. Regular audits and patient feedback loops can be instrumental.

**Influence on Staff Satisfaction and Retention:**
1. **Clear Role Delineation**: A well-defined organizational structure ensures that roles and responsibilities are clear, reducing ambiguities and overlaps, thus enhancing job satisfaction.
2. **Employee Engagement**: Organizations that involve staff in decision-making processes tend to have higher staff satisfaction. This is often a feature of flat or team-based designs.
3. **Opportunities for Growth**: Organizational structures that prioritize continuous learning and professional development often see higher staff retention rates.
4. **Communication Channels**: Effective communication mechanisms, often overseen by governance, can significantly influence staff morale. When employees feel heard and valued, satisfaction often surges.

**Strategies to Ensure High-Quality Patient Care and Staff Satisfaction:**
1. **Continuous Training**: Regular training sessions keep the staff updated on the latest in clinical care, ensuring that patients receive top-notch services.
2. **Feedback Mechanisms**: Implementing robust feedback systems for both patients and staff can be instrumental. For staff, it can shed light on areas of dissatisfaction, while for patients, it provides insights into care quality.
3. **Invest in Technology**: Adopting advanced healthcare technologies, like Electronic Health Records (EHR) or telehealth platforms, can streamline operations, improve patient care, and reduce staff frustrations stemming from outdated systems.

4. **Promote Interdisciplinary Collaboration**: Encouraging departments and specialties to collaborate can enhance patient care by providing comprehensive services and also boost staff morale as they learn from each other.
5. **Wellness Initiatives**: Recognizing the challenges and stresses of healthcare work, governance can prioritize staff wellness initiatives, which can improve overall job satisfaction and indirectly benefit patient care.

*Real-world example*: A renowned hospital, noticing a spike in staff turnover and a dip in patient satisfaction scores, decided to revamp its governance and organizational structure. They shifted to a team-based design, introduced regular inter-departmental meetings, and invested heavily in staff training. They also set up a digital feedback system where patients and staff could voice concerns or suggestions. Over the subsequent years, the hospital saw a considerable drop in staff turnover and a significant rise in patient satisfaction scores. This case underscores how closely intertwined governance decisions, organizational design, and care outcomes can be.

# Leadership:

**Evolution of Leadership Theories in Healthcare**

Over time, leadership theories have evolved to better accommodate the unique dynamics and challenges of the healthcare industry. Initially, leadership in healthcare mirrored traditional hierarchical models seen in other industries, with an emphasis on autocratic or transactional leadership. As healthcare evolved to become more patient-centered and collaborative, so too did the leadership styles to accommodate these shifts.

1. **Autocratic Leadership**: Historically, the healthcare system leaned heavily on autocratic leadership. Decisions were made by senior leaders with little input from subordinates. This top-down approach was believed to be efficient but sometimes lacked in fostering innovation or staff morale.
2. **Transformational Leadership**: By the late 20th century, there was a shift towards transformational leadership. This style motivates and inspires staff to work collaboratively towards a shared vision. Given the interdependent nature of healthcare roles – from doctors and nurses to ancillary staff – this style promotes better team cohesion and patient-centered care.
3. **Servant Leadership**: More recently, servant leadership has gained traction in healthcare. This style emphasizes leaders serving their teams, ensuring they have the resources and support needed to excel in their roles. It aligns well with the healthcare ethos of serving patients.
4. **Shared Leadership**: Recognizing the expertise that each healthcare professional brings, shared leadership promotes decision-making at all levels. It's particularly effective in multidisciplinary teams where varied expertise is essential for holistic patient care.

**Impact of Leadership Styles on Nursing Practices and Outcomes**

Different leadership styles can have profound impacts on nursing practices and, consequently, patient outcomes:

1. **Autocratic Leadership:** Can lead to quick decision-making in crises but may stifle creativity and reduce staff morale if used excessively.
2. **Transformational Leadership:** Enhances job satisfaction, fosters professional development, and is linked to improved patient satisfaction. Nurses are motivated to exceed expectations and provide exceptional patient care.
3. **Servant Leadership:** Improves team dynamics and staff retention. When nurses feel supported, they are better equipped to provide optimal patient care.
4. **Shared Leadership:** Fosters a culture of continuous improvement and accountability. When nurses have a say in decisions, they feel a greater sense of ownership and commitment to positive patient outcomes.

## Historical Figures in Nursing with Distinct Leadership Styles

1. **Florence Nightingale:** Often called the founder of modern nursing, Nightingale displayed transformational leadership qualities. She revolutionized nursing practices based on her observations and data, inspiring others with her vision for improved patient care.
2. **Clara Barton:** Exhibiting traits of servant leadership, Barton, the founder of the American Red Cross, dedicated her life to serving others, especially in times of crises like wars.
3. **Virginia Henderson:** As a nurse theorist, Henderson demonstrated shared leadership qualities. She believed in the importance of patient self-sufficiency and the essential role every team member played in achieving this.

These leaders, among many others, have shaped the nursing profession through their unique leadership styles and continue to inspire modern nursing leaders. Their legacies underline the importance of adaptive and effective leadership in healthcare.

## Transformational vs. Transactional Leadership in Healthcare

**Transformational Leadership:**

- **Characteristics:** Transformational leaders inspire and motivate their teams by creating a shared vision for the future. They are focused on team-building, collaboration, and aligning the organization's mission and values to enhance job performance and satisfaction. This style is about creating positive changes and fostering innovation.
- **Application in Healthcare:** Transformational leadership encourages interdisciplinary teamwork. Nurse executives utilizing this style might advocate for cross-functional teams, where nurses, physicians, and other healthcare workers collaborate for improved patient outcomes.

**Transactional Leadership:**

- **Characteristics:** Transactional leaders work through a clear chain of command and a rewards-based system. They set clear roles and responsibilities, expecting subordinates to follow directives in exchange for rewards or avoid penalties. It's based on transactions, often contingent on performance.
- **Application in Healthcare:** This style can be seen in scenarios where strict compliance is crucial, like following medical protocols or standards of care. For instance, a nurse might be rewarded for consistently documenting patient care accurately and on time.

**Potential Impacts of Transformational Leadership on Patient Outcomes:**
1. **Improved Patient Satisfaction:** By promoting teamwork and collaboration, transformational leaders can lead to holistic patient care. This often translates to higher patient satisfaction scores.
2. **Lower Rates of Medical Errors:** With a focus on innovative problem-solving and continuous learning, transformational leaders may drive initiatives that lead to fewer medical mistakes.
3. **Higher Nurse Job Satisfaction:** Satisfied and motivated nursing staff typically equates to better patient care, as they're more invested in positive patient outcomes.
4. **Innovative Care Approaches:** Emphasizing forward-thinking, these leaders might drive the adoption of cutting-edge patient care technologies or methodologies.

**Scenarios Beneficial for Transactional Leadership in Nursing:**
1. **Clinical Audits:** When ensuring every nurse adheres to set clinical guidelines, transactional leadership's clear directives can be beneficial.
2. **Regulatory Compliance:** With ever-evolving healthcare laws and regulations, transactional leadership ensures that all staff members are adhering to current legal mandates.
3. **Emergency Situations:** In high-pressure scenarios where immediate compliance is necessary, the clear chain of command characteristic of transactional leadership can be life-saving.
4. **Training New Staff:** For novice nurses or staff, the clear structure and expectations set by transactional leaders can provide a solid foundational understanding of their roles.

In summary, while transformational leadership fosters innovation and motivation, driving improved patient satisfaction and care quality, transactional leadership's structured approach can be invaluable in specific scenarios, ensuring adherence to crucial protocols and standards. A successful nurse executive will adeptly blend both styles, leveraging their strengths in appropriate scenarios.

**Servant Leadership in Nursing Management:**
**Definition:** Servant leadership focuses on the leader's role as the servant of their team. It prioritizes the needs of the team members, emphasizing empathy, listening, and commitment to supporting and developing each member of the group.
**Application in Nursing:**
1. **Patient-Centric Care:** By advocating for the needs and professional growth of the nursing staff, servant leaders indirectly promote the best possible patient care. A team that feels supported tends to provide superior patient care.
2. **Promotion of Collaborative Environment:** Servant leadership nurtures a culture of collaboration. It encourages the sharing of knowledge and expertise among the team, ensuring the best solutions for patient issues.
3. **Empowerment:** These leaders often empower nurses to take on leadership roles in patient care, fostering professional growth and ensuring patients receive skilled care.

**Situational Leadership in the Context of a Healthcare Crisis:**

**Definition:** Situational leadership theory proposes that leaders adjust their style based on the situation and the development level of their followers. It revolves around directive and supportive dimensions.

**Application in Healthcare Crisis:**
1. **Assessment of Competence and Confidence:** In a crisis, nurse leaders will assess their team's competence and confidence. For instance, during an outbreak of a new disease, some nurses might be knowledgeable about the ailment, while others may not.
2. **Directive Behavior:** In the early stages of a crisis, when procedures and protocols may be unfamiliar, leaders might be more directive, providing specific instructions to ensure patient safety and effective care.
3. **Supportive Behavior:** As the crisis unfolds and team members become more familiar with their roles and responsibilities, leaders shift to a supportive role, offering encouragement, feedback, and facilitating problem-solving.

**Charismatic Leadership Theory and its Implications for Nursing Teams:**

**Definition:** Charismatic leaders inspire and motivate their teams through their personal charisma. They have a magnetic personality, high energy, and a strong commitment to their vision, which they use to inspire their followers.

**Implications for Nursing Teams:**
1. **Enhanced Motivation:** Charismatic leaders can instill a sense of purpose in their nursing teams. Their enthusiasm can be contagious, leading to a motivated and dedicated staff.
2. **Risk of Over-dependence:** While charismatic leaders can be highly effective, there's a risk that teams become too dependent on their energy and vision. In their absence, the team might feel lost or demotivated.
3. **Potential for Ego Conflicts:** Due to their strong personalities, charismatic leaders might occasionally clash with other equally strong-willed team members. It's crucial for these leaders to harness their charisma for the team's benefit, rather than personal glory.

In healthcare, particularly in nursing, leaders must be adaptable, understanding, and flexible. Given the dynamic nature of healthcare environments, it's essential to understand and employ a range of leadership theories effectively, depending on the context and the needs of the nursing team and patients.

**Top Five Leadership Skills Every Nurse Executive Should Possess:**
1. **Strategic Visioning:** Nurse executives should be able to craft and communicate a clear vision for the future of their department or organization. This involves understanding healthcare trends, foreseeing challenges, and strategizing accordingly.
2. **Decision-making:** Being decisive, especially under pressure, is crucial. This involves analyzing data, considering team input, and making choices that best serve patient care and the organization's goals.
3. **Team Building and Motivation:** A nurse executive should foster team spirit, ensuring every member feels valued and motivated. This involves recognizing achievements, providing growth opportunities, and addressing team conflicts proactively.

4. **Financial Acumen:** Nurse executives must understand budgeting, forecasting, and resource allocation to ensure the best patient care while maintaining fiscal responsibility.
5. **Regulatory and Compliance Knowledge:** With healthcare being a heavily regulated industry, understanding and ensuring compliance with local, state, and federal regulations is paramount.

**Emotional Intelligence in Nursing Leadership:**

Emotional intelligence (EI) encompasses self-awareness, self-regulation, motivation, empathy, and social skills. In nursing leadership:

- **Self-awareness** allows leaders to recognize their emotions and understand their impact on decision-making and interactions.
- **Self-regulation** helps in managing disruptive emotions, essential when handling stressful situations or addressing conflicts.
- **Empathy** ensures leaders can understand and consider the feelings and needs of their team, fostering a supportive environment.
- Enhanced EI leads to better **patient-nurse relationships**, as leaders with high EI often promote empathetic care within their teams.

**Relationship Between Communication Skills and Effective Leadership in Nursing:**

Effective communication is the linchpin of successful leadership. In nursing:

- **Clear Instructions:** Whether it's a new hospital protocol or feedback from a recent audit, nurse executives must communicate information concisely and understandably.
- **Active Listening:** Leaders should listen to their team's concerns, ideas, or feedback, ensuring everyone feels heard and valued.
- **Feedback Mechanisms:** Regular constructive feedback helps in professional growth and addresses potential issues before they escalate.
- **Crisis Communication:** During healthcare crises, clear and calm communication can mean the difference between chaos and coordinated care.
- **Facilitating Inter-departmental Communication:** Nurse executives often act as a bridge between nursing staff and other hospital departments, ensuring seamless patient care.

In essence, nursing leadership isn't just about directing; it's about understanding, empathizing, strategizing, and communicating effectively. Nurse executives, equipped with these skills and knowledge, play a pivotal role in shaping the future of patient care and the nursing profession.

**Common Sources of Conflict within Nursing Teams and Strategies to Address Them:**

1. **Resource Allocation:** Limited resources, be it staffing, equipment, or time, can lead to conflicts over their distribution.

*Strategy:* Transparent criteria for resource distribution, regular team meetings to discuss concerns, and continuous review of resource needs.

2. **Role Ambiguity:** Unclear job descriptions or overlapping roles can lead to confusion and disputes over responsibilities.

*Strategy:* Clearly defined job roles, periodic role reviews, and open communication channels for clarifications.

3. **Differences in Values or Perspectives:** Varied backgrounds and experiences can lead to differing views on patient care.

*Strategy:* Encourage a culture of respect, team-building activities, and regular team discussions to understand and appreciate diverse viewpoints.

4. **Communication Breakdown:** Misunderstandings or lack of communication can escalate minor issues.

*Strategy:* Promote open communication, implement regular team huddles, and use tools like SBAR (Situation, Background, Assessment, Recommendation) for clarity.

5. **Personality Clashes:** Sometimes, individual personalities don't gel well, leading to conflicts.

*Strategy:* Team-building activities, rotation of team members, and conflict resolution training.

**Acting as a Mediator in Inter-departmental Conflicts:**

1. **Neutral Ground:** A nurse executive should maintain neutrality, ensuring all parties feel their perspectives are considered without bias.
2. **Facilitate Dialogue:** Create an environment where each department can voice its concerns and viewpoints.
3. **Focus on Common Goals:** Highlight the shared objective – patient care excellence. This can often redirect the focus from departmental issues to patient-centric solutions.
4. **Seek External Mediation:** If internal resolution is challenging, consider an unbiased third party or a professional mediator.
5. **Action Plans:** After understanding the root of the conflict, draft actionable steps to address the issue and ensure all departments are aligned.

**Long-term Implications of Unresolved Conflicts in Healthcare Settings:**

1. **Decreased Patient Care Quality:** Conflicts can distract healthcare professionals from their primary responsibility, potentially leading to mistakes or oversights.
2. **Reduced Staff Morale:** Persistent conflicts create a toxic work environment, reducing job satisfaction and motivation.
3. **Increased Turnover Rates:** Unresolved conflicts can make professionals seek opportunities elsewhere, leading to high turnover and associated costs.
4. **Inefficient Work Processes:** Conflicts often mean teams aren't collaborating effectively, leading to inefficiencies and delays.
5. **Reputation Damage:** Chronic internal conflicts can spill over, potentially damaging the institution's reputation among patients, families, and the broader healthcare community.

In essence, while conflicts are natural in any dynamic setting like healthcare, addressing them proactively and effectively is paramount. Nurse executives play a crucial role in this, ensuring both the well-being of their teams and the optimum care of their patients.

**Decision-Making Process in Nursing Leadership:**

1. **Assessment:** Gathering relevant information and data about the situation. This could involve patient data, staff feedback, or other pertinent facts.
2. **Diagnosis:** Analyzing the information to pinpoint the issue or challenge.

3.  **Planning:** Determining multiple potential solutions, weighing pros and cons, and selecting the most viable solution.
4.  **Implementation:** Executing the chosen solution with precision and monitoring its progress.
5.  **Evaluation:** Reflecting on the outcome and effectiveness of the decision to make any necessary adjustments or improvements in the future.

**Importance:** Sound decision-making ensures optimal patient care, efficient resource utilization, and a harmonious work environment. It upholds the standards of the nursing profession and meets institutional goals.

**Effective Delegation while Maintaining Accountability:**
1.  **Know Your Team:** Understand each team member's skills, training, and capacity. This ensures tasks are assigned to those best equipped to handle them.
2.  **Clear Communication:** Clearly define what needs to be done, expected outcomes, and any relevant deadlines. Ensure the person receiving the task understands and accepts the responsibility.
3.  **Empower but Monitor:** Give your team the autonomy to complete tasks but set checkpoints or periodic reviews to monitor progress.
4.  **Feedback Mechanism:** Create an open channel where staff can communicate challenges or provide updates on task progress.
5.  **Document Delegation:** Maintain records of all tasks delegated, to whom, and their deadlines. This documentation can be pivotal for accountability and future references.

**Pitfalls in Delegation and Avoidance Strategies:**
1.  **Over-delegation:** Overburdening a team member can lead to burnout and mistakes.
*Avoidance:* Regularly assess workload distribution and adjust as necessary.
2.  **Under-delegation:** Not utilizing the full potential of the team can lead to inefficiencies and discontent.
*Avoidance:* Recognize and trust the skills and expertise of your team. Provide opportunities for growth and skill utilization.
3.  **Ambiguous Instructions:** Providing unclear directives can result in task errors.
*Avoidance:* Prioritize clear, concise communication. Use tools and templates if necessary for clarity.
4.  **Mismatch of Skills:** Delegating tasks to those unequipped to handle them can lead to errors and dissatisfaction.
*Avoidance:* Understand the strengths, weaknesses, and training levels of each team member.
5.  **Lack of Follow-Up:** Without monitoring, it's challenging to track the success or failures of a delegated task.
*Avoidance:* Set periodic review checkpoints and maintain an open line of communication.

In the dynamic and demanding field of healthcare, the ability to make informed decisions and delegate efficiently is paramount. These skills not only drive optimal patient care but also ensure a motivated and resourceful nursing team.

**Empowering Teams for Better Patient Care:**
1. **Shared Decision Making:** Engage team members in the decision-making process. Solicit their opinions, listen actively, and incorporate their feedback. When team members feel their input is valued, they're more motivated and committed.
2. **Provide Professional Development Opportunities:** Invest in ongoing training, workshops, and educational sessions. This not only upgrades the skills of the team but also instills a sense of value and growth.
3. **Acknowledge and Reward:** Recognize outstanding work and efforts. Celebrate achievements, both big and small. This not only boosts morale but also encourages a culture of excellence.
4. **Open Communication Channels:** Foster an environment where team members can voice concerns, share ideas, and provide feedback without fear of retribution.
5. **Delegate with Trust:** Entrust tasks based on competency and then trust your team to execute. Avoid micromanaging, but ensure support when needed.

**Key Negotiation Skills for Nurse Executives:**
1. **Active Listening:** Pay full attention, understand the content, and respond thoughtfully. It helps in understanding the underlying concerns or needs of the other party.
2. **Preparation:** Before entering any negotiation, be well-prepared with all relevant facts, data, and potential solutions.
3. **Clear Communication:** Articulate your needs, concerns, and offerings clearly, avoiding ambiguity.
4. **Problem-Solving Attitude:** Approach negotiations as a problem-solving session rather than a competition. This promotes collaboration.
5. **Emotional Intelligence:** Recognize and understand emotions, both yours and others', to guide your thinking and behavior. This helps in building rapport and trust.
6. **Patience:** Sometimes, negotiations take time. Patience can help you avoid making hasty decisions.

**Scenarios where Negotiation is Pivotal in Nursing Leadership:**
1. **Resource Allocation:** You're in a situation where the hospital budget is tight, and you need to negotiate for necessary equipment or more staffing with senior management.
2. **Conflict Resolution:** Two nurses have a disagreement about a care plan for a patient. As a leader, you might need to mediate and negotiate a solution that respects both views while ensuring optimal patient care.
3. **Inter-Departmental Collaboration:** Suppose radiology and nursing are clashing over the scheduling of patient scans. A nurse leader may need to negotiate with the radiology department head to arrive at a mutually beneficial solution.
4. **Contract Negotiations:** Whether it's negotiating contracts for new hires, vendors, or union agreements, nurse executives play a crucial role in ensuring terms are favorable for both the institution and the staff.
5. **Policy Implementation:** When introducing a new policy or changing an existing one, nurse leaders may need to negotiate with staff to ensure understanding, buy-in, and smooth implementation.

Empowering nursing teams and possessing adept negotiation skills are invaluable assets for nurse executives. They play a significant role in not only enhancing patient care but also fostering a positive, collaborative, and efficient work environment.

**Role of Nurse Executives in Driving Change Within Healthcare Organizations:**
1. **Vision Setting:** Nurse executives are often responsible for visualizing and defining the direction of change, ensuring it aligns with the overarching goals of the healthcare organization.
2. **Stakeholder Engagement:** Engaging physicians, nurses, administrative staff, and even patients is pivotal. Nurse executives play a role in bringing all these stakeholders onboard, ensuring they understand the reasons for change and its potential benefits.
3. **Resource Management:** Change often requires allocating resources differently – whether it's finances, manpower, or technology. Nurse executives decide on these allocations based on the priority of the changes.
4. **Policy and Procedure Development:** To drive change, existing policies and procedures might need adjustments. Nurse executives are instrumental in drafting, revising, and implementing these.
5. **Monitoring and Evaluation:** Post-implementation, nurse executives measure the success of the change, gather feedback, and make necessary tweaks to ensure continuous improvement.
6. **Training and Education:** They ensure that staff is adequately trained and prepared for the change, facilitating smoother transitions.

**Common Barriers to Change in a Healthcare Context:**
1. **Resistance to Change:** A natural human inclination, many fear the unknown or feel threatened by alterations in their routine or responsibilities.
2. **Communication Breakdown:** Without clear communication about the reasons for and benefits of change, rumors and misinformation can spread.
3. **Resource Limitations:** Financial constraints, limited manpower, or technological barriers can hinder the change process.
4. **Organizational Culture:** If the prevailing culture is risk-averse or set in its ways, introducing change becomes more challenging.
5. **Lack of Leadership Support:** Change can falter without full backing from top management and leaders within the organization.
6. **Inadequate Training:** Staff unprepared for change due to insufficient training can lead to mistakes, frustration, and inefficiencies.
7. **Unclear Objectives:** Without well-defined goals or a clear understanding of the change's purpose, implementation can be misguided or half-hearted.

Real-world application: Consider the implementation of Electronic Health Records (EHRs) in a hospital setting. A nurse executive would play a pivotal role in this change – from selecting the right EHR system, allocating resources, training the nursing staff, to troubleshooting post-implementation issues. Barriers might include resistance from older staff unfamiliar with technology, budgetary constraints, or issues integrating the EHR with other existing systems. By understanding and anticipating these barriers, a nurse executive can strategize effectively, ensuring the change brings about improved patient care and streamlined operations.

**Evidence-Based Strategies for Implementing Change in Nursing Practices:**
1. **Plan-Do-Study-Act (PDSA) Cycle:** An iterative, four-stage problem-solving model used for improving processes and products.
   - **Plan:** Identify the change, develop a strategy.
   - **Do:** Implement on a small scale.
   - **Study:** Assess the impact and results.
   - **Act:** If successful, implement on a wider scale; if not, refine and restart the process.
2. **Lewin's Change Model:** Comprises three stages:
   - **Unfreeze:** Recognize the need for change and prepare the organization.
   - **Change:** Execute the planned changes.
   - **Refreeze:** Ensure that the changes are solidified and become the new norm.
3. **Kotter's Eight-Step Process:** A detailed step-by-step approach starting from establishing urgency to consolidating gains and producing more change.
4. **Rogers' Diffusion of Innovations Theory:** Focuses on how innovations are adopted within an organization, categorizing adopters as innovators, early adopters, early majority, late majority, or laggards.
5. **Use of Clinical Practice Guidelines:** Utilizing evidence-based guidelines provides a blueprint for integrating the latest research into practice.
6. **Feedback Mechanisms:** Regular feedback from frontline staff provides insights into the efficacy of the change and areas of improvement.

**Strategies to Ensure Stakeholder Buy-In During Organizational Changes:**
1. **Transparent Communication:** Clearly articulate the need for change, its benefits, and its alignment with the organization's mission and values.
2. **Inclusive Decision-making:** Engage stakeholders in the change process, allowing them to voice their concerns and provide insights.
3. **Tailored Messaging:** Different stakeholders have different priorities. Tailor communication to address the unique needs and concerns of each group.
4. **Education and Training:** Equip stakeholders with the knowledge and tools they need to navigate and embrace the change.
5. **Showcase Early Wins:** Highlighting initial successes can garner more support and increase momentum.
6. **Feedback Loops:** Create mechanisms where stakeholders can provide feedback and express their concerns during the change process.
7. **Visible Leadership Support:** Visible endorsement and involvement of top leaders can significantly influence stakeholder buy-in.
8. **Address Resistance:** Identify and address sources of resistance. This might include additional training, resources, or simply more detailed explanations.

Real-world application: Suppose a hospital is transitioning to a new patient care model. Using evidence-based strategies like PDSA can help in piloting the model in specific departments. Nurse leaders can hold town hall meetings for transparent communication, involve staff in decision-making via committees, offer training sessions, and share success stories from the pilot department to ensure stakeholder buy-in across the entire institution.

**Psychological Roots of Resistance Among Healthcare Professionals:**

1. **Loss of Control:** Changes can sometimes make professionals feel that they're losing their autonomy or ability to control their work environment.
2. **Fear of the Unknown:** Humans inherently fear what they don't know. If changes aren't clearly communicated, it can result in apprehension.
3. **Perceived Threat to Job Security:** Professionals may fear that the changes could make their roles redundant.
4. **Loss of Identity:** Established routines can form a part of one's professional identity. Changes can disrupt this, leading to resistance.
5. **Fear of Failure:** A shift might entail learning new skills. The fear of not being able to adapt can cause professionals to resist.
6. **Peer Pressure:** If influential team members resist, others might follow suit, even if they don't personally oppose the change.
7. **Past Resentments:** Past initiatives that didn't pan out can make professionals skeptical about new ones.

**Effective Strategies for Addressing and Mitigating Resistance in Nursing Teams:**

1. **Transparent Communication:** Make sure everyone understands the reasons for the change, the benefits, and the process.
2. **Involve Them in the Process:** Seek input from those affected by the change. Their front-line experience can provide invaluable insights.
3. **Training and Support:** Offer ample opportunities for training and provide resources to help them navigate the transition.
4. **Address Concerns Directly:** Open forums, Q&A sessions, and one-on-one meetings can be venues where concerns are heard and addressed.
5. **Pilot Programs:** Test changes on a small scale. This gives a tangible demonstration of what to expect and can assuage some fears.
6. **Recognize and Reward:** Acknowledge those who are leading the way and adapting well to the changes.
7. **Peer Champions:** Identify and engage influential team members who support the change. Their endorsement can be instrumental in swaying others.
8. **Consistent Feedback:** Regular check-ins can help identify pockets of resistance and address them promptly.

Example: Consider a hospital implementing a new electronic health record (EHR) system. Nurses, having used the old system for years, might resist the new EHR due to concerns about its complexity or the time it'd take to master it. The nurse executive, aware of this potential resistance, can initiate hands-on training sessions, select a few nurses to pilot the system and provide feedback, and have regular open forums addressing any concerns. Over time, as nurses become acquainted with the new EHR, resistance wanes, especially when they see the system's benefits firsthand and receive support throughout the transition.

**Measuring the Success of Implemented Changes by Nurse Executives:**

1. **Key Performance Indicators (KPIs):** Establish KPIs related to the desired outcomes of the change. For instance, if the change involved implementing a new patient care protocol, one could monitor patient recovery rates, length of hospital stay, or readmission rates.
2. **Surveys and Questionnaires:** Distribute these to staff and patients to gauge satisfaction levels and areas of concern post-change.
3. **Observational Audits:** By directly observing clinical practices, nurse executives can assess whether changes are being adopted and applied correctly.
4. **Data Analytics:** With the rise of electronic health records and digital tools, nurse executives can rely on data analytics to derive insights. For instance, an increase in patient throughput might indicate a successful change in workflow.
5. **Financial Metrics:** Evaluating the financial implications of a change, such as cost savings, increased revenue, or return on investment, can offer insights into its success.
6. **Quality and Safety Metrics:** Monitor rates of incidents, errors, or adverse events. A decrease might indicate successful change implementation.
7. **Staff Retention and Turnover:** Changes that improve the work environment can lead to increased staff retention, while those that don't might see a rise in turnover.

**Importance of Feedback Loops in Evaluating the Effects of Change in Healthcare Settings:**

Feedback loops are critical in the dynamic environment of healthcare for several reasons:

1. **Continuous Improvement:** By constantly receiving feedback, healthcare settings can iteratively refine and enhance changes to optimize results.
2. **Identifying Unintended Consequences:** All changes, even those well-planned, can have unforeseen outcomes. Feedback loops help identify these early on.
3. **Stakeholder Engagement:** Regular feedback involves everyone affected by the change, making them feel valued and heard. This can boost morale and buy-in.
4. **Reinforcing Desired Behaviors:** When staff members receive positive feedback for adapting to changes, it reinforces those behaviors, making the new practices more likely to stick.
5. **Adaptability:** In an ever-evolving field like healthcare, feedback loops ensure that practices remain relevant and effective in the face of new challenges or information.
6. **Transparency and Trust:** An open channel for feedback promotes transparency. When staff members see their feedback being acted upon, it builds trust in leadership.

For instance, after a change in medication administration protocols, a nurse executive might set up monthly feedback sessions for the first six months. If nurses report recurring issues with the new protocol, adjustments can be made promptly. Conversely, positive feedback can be used to showcase success stories and further promote the change. Such feedback loops ensure that the change process remains fluid and responsive to real-world challenges, ultimately leading to better patient outcomes and staff satisfaction.

**Significance of Succession Planning in Nursing Leadership:**
1. **Ensuring Continuity:** Succession planning is vital to ensure that the nursing department or healthcare organization does not experience a leadership vacuum when current leaders retire or leave. It ensures that essential leadership roles are always filled with competent individuals.
2. **Preserving Institutional Knowledge:** Experienced nurse leaders possess vast amounts of institutional knowledge. Succession planning helps transfer this knowledge to the next generation of leaders.
3. **Maintaining and Enhancing Patient Care:** Stable leadership ensures that patient care standards are maintained or even improved. A sudden leadership void can lead to disruptions in care delivery.
4. **Staff Morale and Retention:** Consistent leadership transition promotes a sense of stability among staff, boosting morale and aiding in retention.
5. **Strategic Goal Achievement:** Long-term goals often span the tenures of several leaders. Succession planning ensures that these goals continue to be pursued consistently, regardless of leadership changes.

**Methods to Ensure a Smooth Leadership Transition:**
1. **Identification of Potential Leaders:** Use competency assessments, performance evaluations, and leadership potential metrics to identify staff members who can be groomed for leadership roles.
2. **Mentorship Programs:** Pair potential future leaders with current leaders to benefit from their experience and guidance. This not only helps in skill transfer but also in understanding the nuances of leadership roles.
3. **Leadership Training:** Offer formal leadership training programs to those identified for future leadership roles. This can cover areas like strategic planning, conflict resolution, and financial management.
4. **Cross-training:** Ensure potential leaders understand different aspects of the organization. It's beneficial for them to have experience in various departments or roles.
5. **Clear Communication:** When a leadership change is imminent, communicate it clearly and transparently to all staff members to prevent rumors, uncertainty, or resistance.
6. **Feedback Mechanisms:** Encourage feedback from staff during the transition. It can offer insights into areas of improvement and reassure staff that their input is valued.
7. **Documentation:** Ensure that there are clear and updated job descriptions, policy manuals, and operational guidelines. This documentation serves as a reference for incoming leaders.
8. **Establish a Transition Timeline:** Create a clear timeline for the transition, including overlapping periods where both the outgoing and incoming leader work together.
9. **Evaluate the Transition:** After the transition, assess its effectiveness. Look for areas of improvement that can be applied in future succession plans.

For example, a large hospital might anticipate the retirement of its Chief Nursing Officer (CNO) in two years. Using succession planning, they identify a potential replacement a year in advance, allowing the current CNO to mentor the chosen candidate. This ensures when the CNO retires, the new leader is well-prepared to take over with minimal disruption.

**Importance of Continuous Leadership Training for Potential Successors:**
1. **Dynamic Healthcare Landscape:** The healthcare sector is continually evolving, with changes in technology, regulations, patient care methodologies, and more. Continuous leadership training ensures potential successors are always updated and can effectively navigate these changes.
2. **Skill Enhancement:** Leadership demands a wide range of skills, from strategic planning to interpersonal communication. Continuous training refines and broadens these competencies.
3. **Confidence Building:** Continuous training instills confidence in potential successors. When they are better prepared and equipped with the necessary skills, they can step into leadership roles more confidently.
4. **Crisis Management:** Healthcare settings can face crises, from outbreaks to natural disasters. Continuous training in crisis management prepares potential leaders to handle these situations efficiently.
5. **Ensuring Smooth Transitions:** Continuous training ensures that potential successors are always ready to step in, leading to smoother transitions during unplanned leadership changes.
6. **Stakeholder Trust:** Stakeholders, be it staff, patients, or external partners, have more trust in leaders who are well-trained and updated. It enhances the credibility of the leadership.
7. **Driving Innovation:** Continual learning can inspire potential leaders to think innovatively and bring fresh perspectives and solutions to ongoing challenges.

**Mentorship as a Method for Succession Planning in Nursing:**
1. **Skill Transfer:** Mentorship provides a platform where the mentor, often an experienced leader, can directly transfer skills and knowledge to the mentee. This one-on-one guidance is often more impactful than generic training programs.
2. **Cultural Transmission:** Beyond skills, mentors can also impart the organizational culture, values, and traditions to the mentees. This ensures continuity in the organizational ethos.
3. **Safe Environment for Query Resolution:** Mentees can openly discuss challenges, doubts, and areas of concern with their mentors, receiving personalized advice and solutions.
4. **Networking:** Mentors can introduce mentees to vital networks within and outside the organization, facilitating broader exposure and better understanding of the healthcare landscape.
5. **Feedback Loop:** Continuous feedback from mentors helps mentees identify areas of improvement and grow faster in their roles.

6. **Career Development:** A mentor can guide the mentee in charting out a clear career path, helping them understand the stepping stones to leadership.
7. **Addressing Gaps:** Mentorship can be tailored to address specific gaps in the mentee's knowledge or skills, ensuring a more focused and effective learning process.

For instance, a senior nurse leader mentoring a junior nurse can share experiences of managing complex patient cases, dealing with team conflicts, or navigating hospital bureaucracy. Such insights, which might not be available in formal training programs, can be invaluable for the mentee's growth. The bond formed during mentorship often lasts throughout careers, with the mentor continuing to guide, advise, and support the mentee, even as they ascend leadership roles.

Case Study 1: Transformational Leadership in a Nursing Scenario

Background: Nurse Laura had recently been promoted as the Nursing Manager of the Intensive Care Unit (ICU) at City Hospital. The ICU was facing high staff turnover, low morale, and patient complaints were on the rise.

Action: Laura introduced regular team meetings where everyone, from the newest nurse to the most experienced, was encouraged to share ideas for improvement. She recognized and rewarded innovative ideas and took a personal interest in the professional development of her staff.

Laura introduced mentoring programs, pairing experienced nurses with newer ones. She actively sought feedback, and instead of penalizing mistakes, she turned them into learning opportunities.

Outcome: Within a year, staff turnover had reduced significantly. Nurses began to take initiatives, like developing protocols for specific procedures, which enhanced patient care. The ICU saw a decline in patient complaints, and the morale of the unit improved drastically.

Case Study 2: Challenges of Change Management in Nursing

Background: At Riverdale Hospital, the administration decided to implement a new Electronic Health Record (EHR) system. Nurse Jane, the Nurse Leader, was responsible for ensuring her department's smooth transition.

Challenges: Initial training sessions were met with resistance. Many nurses, especially those who had been in the profession for a long time, found the new system confusing and time-consuming. There was a lot of apprehension and a fear of making mistakes.

Action: Jane acknowledged the concerns of her team. She organized additional hands-on training sessions tailored to different experience levels. She set up a system where nurses could buddy up, with those proficient in the EHR assisting those struggling. Jane also liaised with the IT department to make specific modifications to the system, making it more user-friendly for the nursing staff.

Outcome: The transition to the new EHR system was slower than anticipated, but with fewer hiccups. The nurses felt supported, and the 'buddy' system fostered teamwork and camaraderie.

Case Study 3: Succession Planning in Healthcare

Background: St. Luke's Hospital had a visionary Chief Nursing Officer (CNO), Dr. Emily. Knowing she would retire in five years, she wanted to ensure that her successor would carry forward her vision and ensure stability.

Action: Dr. Emily identified potential leaders within her team and began a structured mentorship program. She involved them in strategic planning, decision-making processes, and exposed them to board meetings and interactions with other department heads. She also sent these potential leaders to leadership development courses.

Three years into her plan, one of the potential successors, Nurse Mike, showed exceptional promise. Dr. Emily then began working closely with Mike, involving him in higher-level decisions and even representing the nursing department in her absence.

Outcome: When Dr. Emily retired, Nurse Mike was appointed as the new CNO. The transition was seamless. Mike's earlier involvement in strategic planning meant he was already aware of the hospital's future plans and was prepared to take the reins. The nursing department didn't face the instability that often comes with leadership changes.

# **Communication and Relationship Building:**

**Communication Theories Relevant to Nursing Leadership**
- **Sender-Receiver Model:** At its core, communication involves a sender, a message, and a receiver. The sender encodes a message, the receiver decodes it, and feedback completes the loop. For nurse executives, understanding this model is crucial. For instance, when conveying new policies, ensuring clarity (encoding) and seeking feedback (decoding) is vital to understand if the message was correctly received.
- **Berlo's SMCR Model:** David Berlo's Source-Message-Channel-Receiver (SMCR) Model delves deeper. It underscores the importance of source (nurse executive) skills, attitudes, knowledge, and socio-cultural system. An executive with strong communication skills using the appropriate channel (e.g., face-to-face for sensitive issues) enhances effective communication.

**Transactional vs. Transformational Communication in Nursing**

- **Transactional Communication:** It's based on linear exchanges - directives, orders, or simple information sharing. For example, a nurse executive might inform staff of a policy change. It's straightforward and often one-directional. However, it can sometimes feel impersonal.
- **Transformational Communication:** Here, communication is about inspiring, motivating, and creating a vision. A nurse executive employing this approach doesn't just announce a change but involves the team in understanding the reasons, benefits, and the bigger picture. It's dialogic, promoting two-way interaction, and often leads to deeper understanding and commitment.

Consider this example: Instead of merely announcing a new scheduling system (transactional), an executive can share the envisioned benefits, solicit feedback, and foster a shared vision of efficient patient care and work-life balance (transformational).

## Relevance of Non-verbal Communication for Nurse Executives

Non-verbal cues encompass facial expressions, body language, gestures, and even tone of voice. For nurse executives:

- **Building Trust:** Authentic facial expressions, such as genuine smiles or empathetic looks, can build trust within the team. Maintaining eye contact, for instance, can convey sincerity and attentiveness.
- **Detecting Discrepancies:** By observing non-verbal cues, an executive can detect if a team member says they're fine, but their body language suggests otherwise, indicating potential issues needing addressing.
- **Enhancing Feedback:** When providing feedback, non-verbal cues like a reassuring pat or open posture can ease potential defensiveness, ensuring the message is received positively.

Consider a real-world scenario: A nurse executive observes a team member looking distracted during a meeting. Instead of ignoring it or making assumptions, the executive later approaches the individual in private, using open body language to convey approachability and concern, fostering an environment where the team member feels safe to communicate any issues.

In essence, mastering both verbal and non-verbal communication techniques enables nurse executives to lead more effectively, ensuring not just information dissemination but fostering environments of trust, motivation, and collaboration.

## Active Listening in Nursing

Active listening is a crucial skill in the realm of nursing and especially for nurse leaders. This technique involves fully concentrating, understanding, responding, and then remembering what the other person is saying. It's an intentional act that demands focus and commitment to the conversation.

1. **Importance for Nurse Leaders**: Nurse leaders often find themselves at the crossroads of administrative decisions and bedside care. Active listening ensures that they can:
   - Understand the concerns, challenges, and needs of their staff.
   - Build trust and rapport with team members.
   - Make informed decisions that consider multiple perspectives.

2. **Impact on Patient Care**: When nurse leaders practice active listening:
   - They can better understand patient feedback and concerns, leading to more tailored care plans.
   - It facilitates a more open and trusting relationship between patients and healthcare providers.
3. **Team Dynamics**: Teams feel valued and understood when leaders actively listen to them. This:
   - Fosters a more collaborative environment.
   - Reduces misunderstandings or miscommunications.
   - Enhances team cohesion and morale.

## Effective Communication Tools in Healthcare

Communication in healthcare has seen a significant evolution, especially with the advent and progression of technology.

1. **Electronic Health Records (EHRs)**: EHRs allow for seamless documentation, storage, retrieval, and sharing of patient information. They ensure that every healthcare professional involved in a patient's care has access to the same data, promoting continuity of care.
2. **Telemedicine Platforms**: With the increase in remote care, telemedicine platforms facilitate video consultations, ensuring care delivery even from a distance.
3. **Secure Messaging Platforms**: Healthcare professionals can discuss patient care in real-time, ensuring immediate resolution of queries or concerns.
4. **Patient Portals**: These allow patients to view their medical records, book appointments, and communicate with their healthcare providers, fostering patient involvement and autonomy.

## Relationship Management Strategies for Nurse Executives

For nurse executives, relationship management is pivotal in creating a harmonious and efficient working environment.

1. **Open Door Policy**: Nurse executives should foster an environment where team members feel comfortable sharing their concerns, ideas, or feedback.
2. **Regular Check-ins**: Whether through team meetings or one-on-ones, regular interactions can gauge team morale and address any potential issues proactively.
3. **Professional Development Opportunities**: Offering opportunities for growth and learning shows team members that their professional advancement is a priority.
4. **Conflict Resolution Skills**: Being equipped to handle disputes and ensuring fair resolutions promotes a positive team environment.
5. **Recognition and Appreciation**: Regularly acknowledging and rewarding good work boosts team morale and motivation.

By implementing these relationship management strategies, nurse executives can build stronger, more cohesive teams, ultimately leading to improved patient outcomes and a more efficient healthcare delivery system.

## Therapeutic Relationships in Nursing

Therapeutic relationships in nursing are foundational to patient care. These relationships are characterized by trust, respect, and professional intimacy, ensuring the patient's needs are at the forefront. Principles central to building these relationships include:

- **Empathy**: Actively trying to understand the patient's feelings and perspectives.
- **Consistency**: Reliable and predictable care fosters trust.
- **Boundaries**: Recognizing and maintaining professional boundaries ensures the relationship remains therapeutic.
- **Patient Autonomy**: Respecting and promoting patients' rights to make decisions about their care.

**Nurse Executives and Therapeutic Relationships**: Nurse executives play a pivotal role in fostering environments where therapeutic relationships thrive. They:

- Model therapeutic communication and behavior for their teams.
- Advocate for resources, such as continuing education on therapeutic communication.
- Promote policies and practices that prioritize patient-centered care.

## Interdisciplinary Collaboration Dynamics

Interdisciplinary collaboration entails multiple healthcare professionals from diverse disciplines working jointly to provide comprehensive patient care. For collaboration to be successful:

- **Mutual Respect**: Recognizing the unique skills and expertise of each discipline.
- **Open Communication**: Facilitating open channels for feedback and dialogue.
- **Shared Goals**: Ensuring all teams align with the primary goal of improved patient outcomes.

**Nurse Leaders as Bridges**: Nurse leaders are pivotal in interdisciplinary collaboration. They:

- Facilitate effective communication between teams.
- Understand and can articulate the roles of various departments, ensuring efficient resource allocation.
- Advocate for nursing perspectives in decision-making forums, ensuring that patient care remains central.

## Conflict Sources and Resolution Strategies

Within nursing teams, conflicts can arise due to:

- **Differing Clinical Opinions**: Variations in training or experience can lead to differing views on patient care.
- **Resource Constraints**: Limited resources can lead to competition and disagreements on allocations.
- **Personal Conflicts**: Differences in personalities or communication styles can lead to misunderstandings.

**Strategies for Nurse Executives**:

- **Active Listening**: Understand the root causes of conflicts before implementing solutions.
- **Conflict Resolution Training**: Equip teams with skills to handle disagreements proactively.
- **Team-Building Activities**: Foster team cohesion and mutual respect.

- **Open Communication Channels**: Promote an environment where team members feel comfortable voicing concerns or disagreements.
- **Regular Check-ins**: By consistently gauging team dynamics, nurse executives can address budding issues before they escalate.

In sum, the realm of nursing leadership, especially for nurse executives, is complex. It's an interplay of interpersonal skills, a deep understanding of healthcare dynamics, and a commitment to patient-centered care. The strategies and principles touched upon are crucial for ANCC nurse executive aspirants to grasp and internalize.

## Significance of Promoting Diversity and Inclusivity in Nursing

Diversity and inclusivity in nursing go beyond mere representation. They are foundational elements that drive excellence in patient care. Here's why:

1. **Reflecting Patient Demographics**: As patient populations become increasingly diverse, a corresponding nursing team can better understand and cater to specific cultural, linguistic, and social needs.
2. **Holistic Care**: Diverse teams bring varied perspectives, experiences, and knowledge. This diversity can lead to more comprehensive and holistic care solutions, catering to a broader range of patient needs.
3. **Improved Patient Satisfaction**: Patients often feel more comfortable and understood when cared for by professionals who share or respect their cultural, ethnic, or linguistic backgrounds, leading to better satisfaction scores and outcomes.
4. **Innovation and Problem Solving**: Diverse teams tend to be more innovative. Different backgrounds bring various problem-solving approaches, leading to innovative solutions.
5. **Workforce Sustainability**: An inclusive environment attracts and retains talent. When nurses feel respected and included, there's a higher likelihood they'll remain committed to the organization.

## Strategies for Nurse Leaders to Foster an Inclusive Practice Environment

1. **Education and Training**: Offer regular diversity and cultural competence training sessions. Ensure these sessions are practical, with actionable steps that nurses can integrate into their daily routines.
2. **Hiring Practices**: Revise hiring protocols to minimize biases and promote diversity. This might include blind application reviews or employing diverse hiring panels.
3. **Mentorship Programs**: Pairing newer nurses from underrepresented backgrounds with established mentors can aid in retention and professional development.
4. **Open Dialogue**: Create a safe space for nurses to discuss diversity and inclusion-related topics. This could be in the form of regular team meetings or feedback sessions.
5. **Celebrate Diversity**: Recognize and celebrate diverse cultural events, holidays, and observances. This not only educates but also fosters a sense of belonging.
6. **Zero Tolerance for Discrimination**: Have a clear and enforceable policy against any form of discrimination. Ensure that all team members are aware of it, and understand the consequences of violating it.

7. **Feedback Mechanisms**: Implement anonymous feedback mechanisms, allowing staff to voice concerns about inclusivity and diversity without fear of reprisal.
8. **Resource Groups**: Support or establish employee resource groups for underrepresented nurses. These groups can provide peer support and play a pivotal role in policy recommendations.
9. **Leadership Representation**: Strive to have diverse representation in leadership roles. This sends a strong message about the organization's commitment to inclusivity.

In conclusion, diversity and inclusivity in nursing are not just ethical imperatives; they're vital for the delivery of high-quality patient care. Nurse leaders play a crucial role in weaving these principles into the very fabric of healthcare settings, ensuring that both staff and patients reap the benefits.

### Case Studies on Celebrating Diversity in Nursing Teams

*Case 1: Enhancing Linguistic Care* A hospital located in a diverse urban area observed a growing number of non-English speaking patients, particularly those speaking Spanish and Arabic. In response, the nursing team, which already had a few bilingual members, began a 'Language Champion' initiative. Nurses proficient in these languages took additional training to be able to translate medical terms and engage more thoroughly with patients. The outcome? Reduction in miscommunication-related incidents, improved patient satisfaction, and increased adherence to medical recommendations.

*Case 2: Cultural Sensitivity in Pediatric Care* In a pediatric unit of a large hospital, nursing staff often encountered diverse cultural beliefs about medical care and child-rearing. When a nurse of Southeast Asian descent joined the team, she introduced practices in line with those cultural beliefs, such as traditional postpartum practices. By incorporating these practices alongside standard care, the team observed improved postpartum recovery among mothers from that demographic, and increased trust between families and healthcare providers.

### Challenges in Implementing Inclusive Practices and Solutions

1. **Resistance to Change:**
   - *Challenge*: Long-standing team members may resist new practices or view them as unnecessary.
   - *Solution*: Regular diversity training and inclusion workshops can illustrate the benefits and importance of diverse practices. Sharing success stories, like the ones above, can help in winning over skeptics.

2. **Unconscious Bias:**
   - *Challenge*: Even well-meaning professionals may have unconscious biases that influence their actions.
   - *Solution*: Incorporate regular unconscious bias training and encourage self-reflection. Offer resources, like seminars or online courses, on understanding and combating these biases.

3. **Resource Allocation:**
   - *Challenge*: There might be a perception that focusing on diversity and inclusion takes resources away from other crucial areas.

- *Solution*: Demonstrate that inclusive practices improve patient care and can even lead to operational efficiencies in the long run. Present data and case studies to make the case.
4. **Retention of Diverse Talent**:
    - *Challenge*: Even after hiring a diverse nursing team, retaining them can be a challenge if they feel isolated or unsupported.
    - *Solution*: Create mentorship programs, diversity councils, and resource groups to offer support. Ensure that the organizational culture is not just diverse, but genuinely inclusive.
5. **Overemphasis on One Aspect of Diversity**:
    - *Challenge*: In an effort to become more diverse, organizations might focus too much on one aspect, e.g., race, and ignore others, e.g., age or disability.
    - *Solution*: Take a comprehensive view of diversity, ensuring that all voices, regardless of their background, are heard and valued.

In sum, for nurse executives, the path to inclusivity requires consistent commitment, flexibility in approach, and an understanding that diversity is a multi-faceted asset. While challenges are inevitable, the potential benefits in terms of patient care, team cohesion, and overall healthcare outcomes are undeniable.

# Professional Practice and Delivery of Care:

Let's break down the differences and advantages of two prevalent Models of Care in Nursing: **Patient-Centered Care** and **Team Nursing**.
**Patient-Centered Care:**
**Definition**: Patient-Centered Care revolves around tailoring healthcare services to individual patient needs, values, and preferences. It champions active involvement of patients in their own care processes.
**Advantages**:
1. **Personalized Care**: Recognizes individual patient needs, ensuring that interventions are tailored accordingly.
2. **Improved Patient Satisfaction**: As patients are active participants in their care, they often report higher levels of satisfaction.
3. **Enhanced Patient Compliance**: Patients who understand and agree with their care plans are more likely to follow through with treatments.

**Example Scenario**: A 60-year-old diabetic patient is being treated in an outpatient setting. In the patient-centered model, the care team spends time understanding his daily routine, diet, work commitments, and personal beliefs about treatment. Based on this information, they tailor a diabetes management plan specific to his needs, ensuring he understands his role in the management. This approach enhances his adherence to the treatment plan, resulting in better glycemic control.
**Team Nursing:**

**Definition**: Team Nursing is a model where a team of healthcare professionals, led by a nurse, collaborates to provide care to a group of patients. The team can consist of RNs, LPNs, nursing aides, and sometimes specialists, all delivering care under the direction and delegation of the lead nurse.

**Advantages**:

1. **Efficiency**: By dividing tasks among team members according to their competence and scope of practice, care can be delivered more efficiently.
2. **Holistic Care**: The collaboration of various professionals ensures that the patient receives comprehensive care.
3. **Shared Responsibility**: Challenges and issues in patient care are tackled collaboratively, reducing the burden on any single individual.

**Example Scenario**: On a busy orthopedic floor, post-operative patients require various levels of care - wound dressing, physiotherapy, pain management, and patient education about mobility aids. In the team nursing model, the lead nurse coordinates the care. An LPN might handle wound dressings, a nurse's aide assists with patient mobility, and a registered nurse manages pain medication and educates the patient. The combined expertise ensures comprehensive care, leading to quicker recoveries and reduced hospital stays.

**In Conclusion**: While both models have their distinct advantages, the choice largely depends on the healthcare setting, available resources, and specific patient needs. Patient-Centered Care is most effective in scenarios where individualized plans and patient involvement are crucial for optimal outcomes. Team Nursing, on the other hand, is highly beneficial in busy settings or when patient needs are diverse and require a multi-skilled approach.


Care Coordination, at its core, is like the rhythm of a well-conducted orchestra in the vast, bustling domain of healthcare. It ensures that every stakeholder—be it physicians, nurses, specialists, or even the administrative staff—works in harmony to provide seamless, effective patient care.

**Significance of Care Coordination in Nursing**:

- **Reduced Care Fragmentation**: Imagine a patient with multiple conditions, each treated by a different specialist. Without coordination, these treatments might clash or overlook essential elements, resulting in suboptimal patient outcomes. Coordination minimizes this risk.
- **Enhanced Patient Safety**: Effective communication between departments reduces medication errors, misdiagnoses, and repetitive testing.
- **Optimized Resources**: Coordinated care reduces hospital readmissions, unnecessary interventions, and utilizes healthcare resources more efficiently.
- **Improved Patient Satisfaction**: When patients experience a streamlined healthcare journey, their satisfaction and trust in the care system rise.

**Tools and Strategies for Effective Coordination**:

1. **Electronic Health Records (EHR)**: A digital version of a patient's paper chart, EHRs are real-time, patient-centered records that make information available instantly and

securely to authorized users. Nurse executives should champion the adoption and proper use of EHR systems.

2. **Interprofessional Collaborative Practice**: This model encourages different professionals to function cohesively. It's about regular team meetings, interdisciplinary rounds, and co-management of patients.

3. **Standardized Protocols**: Developing and employing standardized care protocols ensures that care delivery remains consistent, irrespective of the provider or setting.

4. **Patient Portals**: These digital tools empower patients to access their health data, communicate with care providers, and schedule appointments, enhancing their involvement and understanding.

**Transition of Care (ToC)**: Transitions are pivotal. It's a handoff, and like in any relay race, a fumbled handoff can have dire consequences. In healthcare, a failed transition can lead to serious patient complications or even mortality.

To ensure optimal ToC:

- **Structured Communication Tools**: SBAR (Situation, Background, Assessment, Recommendation) is an example of a communication tool that standardizes information transfer between professionals, reducing ambiguities.

- **Medication Reconciliation**: This is the process of creating the most accurate list possible of all medications a patient is taking and comparing that list to the physician's admission, transfer, or discharge orders.

- **Follow-up Appointments and Referrals**: Before discharge, scheduling follow-up appointments and referrals ensures continued care.

- **Educate and Engage the Patient**: Before any transition, patients should understand their diagnosis, care plan, and next steps.

**Ensuring Continuity and Safety**: When care coordination and ToC strategies are effectively employed, they act as the threads that stitch the fabric of a patient's healthcare journey. Continuity is maintained as every provider has the full picture, making informed decisions, and ensuring interventions are complementary and not conflicting. Patient safety, on the other hand, is preserved as errors are minimized, potential issues are flagged early, and the patient remains engaged and informed throughout.

To sum it up, think of care coordination as an exquisite dance, and the nurse executive is the choreographer. They ensure each step flows seamlessly into the next, creating a mesmerizing performance—only, in this case, the applause is the enhanced health and well-being of the patient.

Quality Improvement (QI) in nursing is akin to the guiding north star for healthcare organizations, ensuring patient care is consistently moving toward excellence. It's a systematic, continuous effort not just to maintain standards, but to elevate them. It's about rectifying mistakes, anticipating them, and innovating for tomorrow. For a nurse executive, understanding and championing QI is paramount.

**Principles of Quality Improvement in Nursing:**

1. **Patient-Centricity**: Always prioritize patient needs, experiences, and outcomes. Their satisfaction and safety should guide any QI process.
2. **Systematic Approach with Continuous Feedback**: Instead of isolated actions or decisions, QI is a continuous loop of feedback and adjustment.
3. **Team Collaboration**: Everyone, from nurses to physicians to administrative staff, plays a role in QI. Collaboration ensures diverse perspectives, fostering comprehensive solutions.
4. **Evidence-Based Decision Making**: Rely on current scientific evidence, best practices, and updated guidelines to inform QI initiatives.

**Integral QI Processes:**
1. **Assessment**: Regularly evaluate current practices against set benchmarks or standards. This identifies gaps and areas of potential improvement.
2. **Plan-Do-Study-Act (PDSA) Cycle**: A repeated four-stage model used to carry out change:
   - **Plan**: Identify and strategize an improvement.
   - **Do**: Implement the improvement on a small scale.
   - **Study**: Reflect on the results. Was the change beneficial?
   - **Act**: If successful, implement the improvement on a larger scale. If not, reassess and adjust.
3. **Measurement and Analysis**: Constantly gather and evaluate data on performance indicators. Analyze trends and patterns.
4. **Standardization**: Once a new best practice is identified, make it the new standard. Train the team, update protocols, and ensure consistent application.
5. **Feedback Loop**: Encourage feedback from staff and patients. This feedback is invaluable for continuous refinement.

**Tools and Techniques for Nurse Executives:**
1. **Flowcharts**: Visual representations of a process. They help in identifying bottlenecks, redundancies, or lapses in a process.
2. **Root Cause Analysis (RCA)**: A systematic approach used after adverse events to identify the root causes. It digs deeper beyond the apparent reasons to identify underlying issues.
3. **Checklists**: Simple yet effective. They ensure consistency and completeness in executing a task.
4. **Benchmarking**: Compare the practices and outcomes of your organization with top-performing, 'benchmark' organizations to identify gaps and potential strategies for improvement.
5. **Control Charts**: A graphical display of data over time, showing variations in a process. They can help determine if a process is behaving consistently or if there are out-of-control variables.
6. **Baldrige Excellence Framework**: A leadership and performance management framework that focuses on criteria like leadership; strategy; customers; measurement, analysis, and knowledge management; workforce; operations; and results.

7. **Surveys and Feedback Tools**: Tools like the Hospital Consumer Assessment of Healthcare Providers and Systems (HCAHPS) can provide insights into patient satisfaction and areas for improvement.

Nurse executives, by mastering these principles, processes, tools, and techniques, can spearhead QI initiatives in their organizations. Through persistent efforts, they can drive their teams toward delivering care that isn't just adequate, but exemplary. It's about ensuring every patient gets the best, every single time.

Regulatory and Accreditation Compliance in the field of nursing isn't just about crossing t's and dotting i's; it's the safeguard that ensures patient safety, elevates the standard of care, and promotes professionalism within the nursing realm.

**Key Regulations Impacting Nursing Care**:
1. **Nurse Practice Acts (NPA)**: Each state in the U.S. has an NPA which delineates the legal scope of nursing practice. It's an absolute compass for what nurses can and cannot do legally. The NPA covers definitions of nursing, requirements for licensure, and the grounds for disciplinary action against a nurse.
2. **The Joint Commission (TJC)**: An independent, non-profit organization, TJC offers accreditation to hospitals and health care organizations. They have a plethora of standards related to patient care processes, staff competency, and the environment in which care is provided.
3. **The Centers for Medicare & Medicaid Services (CMS)**: CMS establishes conditions that healthcare providers must meet to participate in Medicare and Medicaid. This includes regulations on patient rights, nursing services, and quality assessment and performance improvement.
4. **Occupational Safety and Health Administration (OSHA)**: While not exclusively for nursing, OSHA regulations protect healthcare workers from workplace hazards, ensuring that the environment they work in remains safe.
5. **Health Insurance Portability and Accountability Act (HIPAA)**: This law is about patient privacy, stipulating that health professionals, including nurses, must protect patient health information.
6. **State Board of Nursing**: Each state has its board which creates rules and regulations for duly licensed nurses in their jurisdiction.

**Implications on Daily Nursing Practice**:
1. **Guided Practice**: These regulations and compliances dictate the scope and limitations of a nurse's practice. Whether it's the type of medication a nurse can administer, or the kind of medical procedure they can assist with, the guidelines are clear.
2. **Professional Development**: Adherence to these standards often requires continuous education. This ensures nurses are updated with the latest in care standards, tools, and techniques.
3. **Quality of Care**: Meeting regulatory standards directly translates to higher quality care. From patient safety to optimal outcomes, the set standards ensure a consistent level of quality across the board.

4. **Legal and Ethical Implications**: Non-compliance isn't just about penalties or loss of accreditation. It's a breach of trust with patients and might even lead to legal ramifications.
5. **Patient Trust and Confidence**: When patients know they're in a facility that adheres to strict standards, their confidence and trust in the care provided increases manifold.
6. **Interdisciplinary Collaboration**: Regulations often necessitate seamless collaboration between different departments. This holistic approach, where everyone from the physician to the janitorial staff plays a role, improves patient outcomes.
7. **Documentation and Communication**: A significant part of compliance is documentation. Whether it's patient records, drug administration logs, or incident reports, the significance of clear, concise, and thorough documentation cannot be stressed enough.

*Real-World Example*: Consider a scenario where a patient's health information is unintentionally disclosed due to lax privacy measures. This is a breach of HIPAA regulations. Not only does it compromise the patient's trust but can result in hefty fines for the institution and disciplinary action against the involved personnel.

For nurse executives, these regulations aren't just rules to be followed. They're a reflection of the commitment to patient care, professional integrity, and the relentless pursuit of excellence in the nursing field.

Preparing for accreditations and audits is a rigorous process, often requiring meticulous attention to detail and thorough knowledge of standards. Nurse executives play a pivotal role in ensuring that their teams are adequately prepared, ensuring not just compliance, but also the highest level of patient care.

**Steps for Preparation**:
1. **Understand the Standards**: Nurse executives should be intimately familiar with the criteria set by accrediting bodies, be it The Joint Commission (TJC), Magnet Recognition Program, or state-specific agencies.
2. **Regular Self-assessments**: Implement a system of regular self-assessments or mock audits to determine areas of non-compliance and rectify them immediately.
3. **Training and Education**: Ensure all nursing staff undergo continuous training programs that acquaint them with the latest guidelines, practices, and technologies in the field.
4. **Documentation**: Prioritize immaculate record-keeping. Every patient interaction, treatment, and outcome should be thoroughly documented, leaving no room for discrepancies.
5. **Engage the Team**: Involve the entire nursing team in the preparation process. This not only disseminates responsibility but also fosters a collective commitment to achieving the standards.
6. **Resource Allocation**: Ensure that the necessary resources, both human and material, are adequately allocated to meet the required standards.
7. **Environment and Equipment Check**: Ensure all equipment is up-to-date, properly maintained, and calibrated. The environment should be conducive to patient care, considering factors like hygiene, accessibility, and safety.

8. **Feedback Mechanism**: Set up a feedback loop with staff to understand challenges, obstacles, and suggestions. Often, frontline staff can provide invaluable insights that might be overlooked at an administrative level.
9. **Communication**: Maintain open channels of communication with accrediting bodies. This proactive approach can help understand expectations, get clarifications, and even get insights on how to meet certain challenging standards.
10. **Review and Update Policies**: Regularly review institutional policies to ensure they align with current standards, making updates as necessary.

**Primary Elements Auditors and Accreditors Look For:**
1. **Patient Care Quality and Safety**: Are patients receiving care that meets or exceeds standards? Are there protocols to prevent errors or adverse events?
2. **Competency of Staff**: Are nurses and other staff members adequately trained and credentialed?
3. **Environment**: Is the healthcare setting safe, clean, and conducive to patient well-being?
4. **Patient Rights**: Are patients' rights being respected, including informed consent and privacy?
5. **Documentation**: Are patient records accurately and comprehensively maintained?
6. **Continuous Quality Improvement Initiatives**: Is there a commitment to continuous improvement? Are there mechanisms in place for this?
7. **Emergency Protocols**: Are there clear protocols for emergencies, and are staff trained to handle them?

**Benefits of a Proactive Approach:**
1. **Enhanced Patient Care**: Proactively meeting standards means that the level of patient care is always at its best.
2. **Reduced Stress**: Instead of last-minute scrambles, a continual adherence to standards means less stress during the actual audit.
3. **Professional Development**: Regular training sessions and a commitment to excellence contribute to the professional growth of the nursing staff.
4. **Financial Implications**: Avoiding penalties or potential lawsuits stemming from non-compliance can have significant financial implications.
5. **Reputation**: Achieving and maintaining accreditation boosts the reputation of the institution, making it a preferred choice for patients and attracting the best talent in the nursing field.

*Real-World Example*: A hospital in Texas proactively adopted a program where they did monthly mock drills simulating accreditation audits. When the actual accreditation process took place, they were commended for their practices, faced minimal non-compliance issues, and were able to navigate the process smoothly, much to the relief of the staff and benefit of their patients.

In conclusion, for nurse executives, the mantra should be 'always be prepared.' Accreditations and audits shouldn't be events but rather integral parts of the care delivery system.

# Knowledge of the Healthcare Environment:

**Healthcare Economics in Nursing Practice**

**Healthcare Economics** is a study that evaluates how resources are allocated in the healthcare sector. When it comes to nursing practice, understanding these economic principles is crucial, as they influence almost every facet of patient care, from staffing ratios to the availability of medications.

1. **Supply and Demand in Nursing**:
   - **Supply** refers to the available resources, which, in nursing, can include the number of trained nurses, available beds, equipment, medications, and more. For instance, in areas with nursing shortages, the supply is lower than the demand.
   - **Demand** in nursing relates to the need for healthcare services. An aging population or an outbreak of a disease can significantly increase the demand for nursing care.

The intersection of supply and demand dictates many aspects of healthcare, including costs. For example, when there's a shortage of nurses but a high demand for healthcare services, wages may increase to attract more nurses to the profession.

2. **Resource Allocation**:
   - This refers to how various resources, like time, manpower, and equipment, are distributed within a healthcare setting. Effective resource allocation is vital for maximizing patient care quality while staying within budget constraints.
   - In nursing, this could involve decisions like how many patients a nurse is assigned, which tasks are prioritized, or how funds are allocated for training or equipment.

3. **Implications for Nurse Executives**:
   - **Strategic Planning**: Nurse executives must consider the broader economic landscape when making plans for the future. This might include anticipating future shortages, understanding demographic shifts affecting patient needs, or recognizing upcoming policy changes that could affect funding.
   - **Resource Allocation**: Given that resources are often limited, nurse executives must decide how to distribute them most effectively. This requires a deep understanding of both the immediate needs of the patient population and the long-term goals of the institution.
   - **Recruitment and Retention**: If demand for nurses exceeds supply, executives need strategies to recruit and retain staff. This might include offering competitive salaries, professional development opportunities, or other benefits.

In conclusion, healthcare economics profoundly influences nursing by determining how resources are allocated and used. Nurse executives must understand these principles to make informed decisions that optimize patient care outcomes while ensuring the financial sustainability of their institutions.

**Financing and Reimbursement Models:**

1. **Fee-for-Service (FFS):**
   This traditional reimbursement model pays providers based on the number of services they deliver.
   - *Pros*: Straightforward; providers are reimbursed for each service rendered.
   - *Cons*: Can lead to overtreatment or unnecessary procedures, as payment is directly tied to volume.
   - *Impact on Nurse Executives*: Decision-making might emphasize the quantity of care delivered over quality. Resource allocation may lean towards high-revenue-generating procedures.

2. **Capitation:**
   Providers receive a set amount per patient, irrespective of the number of services utilized by that patient.
   - *Pros*: Promotes efficient care and discourages unnecessary procedures.
   - *Cons*: Potential risk of undertreatment to minimize costs.
   - *Impact on Nurse Executives*: Prioritizes proactive patient care and preventive services. Resource allocation may favor general well-being and outreach programs.

3. **Value-Based Reimbursement (VBR):**
   Providers are compensated based on the quality of care they deliver, typically linked to specific performance metrics.
   - *Pros*: Rewards high-quality care, emphasizing best practices and evidence-based treatments.
   - *Cons*: Necessitates comprehensive data tracking and can be intricate to administer.
   - *Impact on Nurse Executives*: Stresses continuous improvement, training, and adherence to best practices. Resource allocation might focus on areas that directly impact quality metrics.

4. **Bundled Payments:**
   Providers receive a consolidated payment for all services linked to a particular treatment or condition over a defined duration.
   - *Pros*: Fosters coordination and efficiency among providers.
   - *Cons*: Administration can be complex; risk arises if care costs exceed the bundled payment.
   - *Impact on Nurse Executives*: Advocates streamlined care pathways and close coordination between departments. Resource allocation considers the entire care episodes.

5. **Global Budgeting:**
   Hospitals or providers receive a fixed sum to address all expenses for a predetermined period, often a year.
   - *Pros*: Defined expenditure limits foster efficiency.
   - *Cons*: Potential budget constraints may hinder flexibility.

- *Impact on Nurse Executives*: Necessitates an expansive view of resource allocation, ensuring equitable distribution while adhering to the budget's limits.

**Implications for Nurse Executives**:

- **Decision-making**: With VBR, there's an accent on quality, potentially prioritizing training and best practices. Conversely, FFS might emphasize high-volume procedures or services.
- **Resource Allocation**: Under capitation or global budgeting, the goal is to curtail costs without compromising care quality. This may lead to investments in preventive care or technology to bolster efficiency.
- **Care Priorities**: Bundled payments could prompt nurse executives to design streamlined care pathways for specific ailments. In contrast, VBR would target conditions or treatments where quality metrics are paramount.

Nurse executives must adeptly traverse this intricate landscape, harmonizing financial viability with the primary objective of unparalleled patient care. The selected reimbursement model profoundly influences care delivery, making an in-depth understanding pivotal for efficacious nursing leadership.

**Budgeting for Nurse Executives**:

**Key Components of a Nursing Department Budget**:

1. **Operational Expenses**: The day-to-day costs associated with running the department. This includes salaries, utility bills, and supplies.
2. **Capital Expenses**: One-time expenses for long-term investments like purchasing equipment or renovating a unit.
3. **Revenue Projections**: Based on billable patient services and other revenue sources, such as grants or donations.
4. **Variable Costs**: Costs that fluctuate depending on patient volume, like medications and medical supplies.
5. **Fixed Costs**: Costs that remain constant irrespective of patient volume, such as salaried personnel or facility rent.
6. **Indirect Costs**: Expenses shared across departments, like hospital-wide marketing or administrative overhead.
7. **Projected Volume**: Estimates of patient counts, services provided, or procedures performed, influencing revenue and variable costs.

**Challenges in the Budgeting Process**:

1. **Predicting the Unpredictable**: Foreseeing exact patient volumes or emergent medical trends can be daunting.
2. **Balancing Act**: Walking the tightrope between financial constraints and ensuring optimal patient care.
3. **Evolving Healthcare Landscape**: Regulatory changes, shifting reimbursement models, and new care standards can alter budgetary needs.
4. **Technology & Innovation Costs**: Staying abreast of medical advancements often necessitates investment in new equipment or training.

5. **Staffing Concerns**: Managing the needs for adequate staffing versus the costs associated with personnel, including potential overtime or agency staffing expenses.

**Best Practices for Aligning Budgets with Objectives & Institutional Goals:**
1. **Collaborative Budgeting**: Engage multiple stakeholders, including clinical staff, to glean frontline insights. After all, the nurse on the floor often knows what's most needed.
2. **Regularly Review and Adjust**: Instead of a static, annual event, consider budgeting as a dynamic, ongoing process. Regular check-ins can help in adjusting for unpredicted costs or revenues.
3. **Leverage Data Analytics**: Utilize technology to predict trends, analyze past spending, and optimize resource allocation. This isn't just about numbers; it's about smartly deciphering what they signify.
4. **Align with Strategic Goals**: Ensure the nursing department's budget ties into the broader hospital or health system's mission, vision, and strategic objectives.
5. **Prioritize Patient Outcomes**: While financial solvency is vital, always position patient care at the forefront. Optimal patient outcomes often align with efficient, cost-effective care in the long run.
6. **Education & Training**: Invest in ongoing education and training for staff. Well-trained staff can lead to better patient outcomes, which can influence reimbursement, especially in value-based models.

**Real-World Application**: Consider a scenario where a nursing department identified recurrent patient readmissions for a specific ailment, leading to increased costs and reduced reimbursements. By adjusting the budget to fund a new preventative care initiative, not only can they reduce readmissions (and associated costs) but also enhance patient care and satisfaction.

In conclusion, for a nurse executive, budgeting isn't merely about balancing the books. It's a strategic endeavor, marrying fiscal responsibility with the unwavering goal of top-tier patient care. When these align, both the institution and its patients thrive.

**Health Policies: Local, State, and National Levels**
**Evolution of Major Health Policies:**
- **Local Level**: Local health policies often revolve around community health needs, sanitation, local health department functions, and epidemic control. Over time, localities have recognized the importance of addressing social determinants of health, leading to policies addressing housing, food access, and environmental health.
- **State Level**: States have been instrumental in the evolution of Medicaid, public health campaigns, licensure regulations, and state-funded health programs. Many states have taken the initiative to expand Medicaid under the Affordable Care Act, leading to wider coverage.
- **National Level**: On a national scale, the progression of health policies can be witnessed in milestones like the creation of Medicare and Medicaid (1965), the Health Maintenance Organization Act (1973), the Children's Health Insurance Program (1997), and the Affordable Care Act (2010).

**Current State:**
- **Local:** Local health policies are increasingly emphasizing community collaboration, particularly given the impact of the COVID-19 pandemic. They're fostering partnerships with local organizations, schools, and businesses to enhance community health.
- **State:** States are navigating the challenges of healthcare access, affordability, and quality. With ongoing debates about Medicaid expansion, states are also grappling with the opioid crisis, mental health, and rural health disparities.
- **National:** The Affordable Care Act remains a pivotal policy, though it faces discussions about revisions or replacements. Prescription drug pricing, Medicare reform, and health equity are also at the forefront.

**Forecast of Potential Shifts:**
- **Local:** Anticipate more grassroots movements leading to local health policy changes, emphasizing preventive care and community-based interventions.
- **State:** Telehealth regulations, mental health parity, and continued Medicaid discussions will likely dominate state agendas.
- **National:** With an aging population, Medicare sustainability will be a topic of debate. Universal healthcare or single-payer systems could also enter discussions, as will topics surrounding health equity and systemic disparities.

**Impact on Nursing Practice and Nurse Executives:**
- **Direct Impacts:**
  - **Scope of Practice:** State-level regulations can define the roles of Nurse Practitioners, Registered Nurses, and Licensed Vocational Nurses.
  - **Staffing Ratios:** Policies may dictate nurse-to-patient ratios, ensuring patient safety.
  - **Education and Licensure:** State boards govern nursing education prerequisites, licensure requirements, and continuing education.
- **Indirect Impacts:**
  - **Reimbursement Models:** National policies influence reimbursement rates, affecting institutional budgets and, by extension, nursing departments.
  - **Technology and Reporting:** Policies around electronic health records or quality reporting can shape how nurses document care and measure outcomes.
- **Responsibilities in Policy Advocacy & Compliance:**
  - **Staying Informed:** Nurse executives must be conversant with ever-evolving health policies to ensure institutional compliance.
  - **Advocacy:** Leveraging their unique frontline perspective, nurse executives can advocate for policies that bolster patient care, nursing practice, and healthcare systems at large.
  - **Implementation & Training:** Once policies are enacted, nurse executives spearhead their implementation, ensuring teams are educated, resources are allocated, and compliance is maintained.

In essence, health policies, whether local, state, or national, intertwine with the nursing realm. Nurse executives, positioned at this intersection, bear the dual mantle of compliance and advocacy, always championing optimal patient care within the broader healthcare tapestry.

**Healthcare Delivery Models: An Exploration**

**1. Fee-for-Service (FFS):**
- **Strengths**: Direct, straightforward payment structure; providers are paid for the specific services they offer.
- **Weaknesses**: Can lead to over-utilization of services; does not necessarily reward quality of care.
- **Influence on Nursing**: Nurses may see a higher volume of patients with a focus on direct interventions over preventive care.
- **Role of Nurse Executives**: Ensure appropriate billing and documentation while emphasizing quality care and ethical service provision.

**2. Managed Care Organizations (MCOs):**
- **Strengths**: Aim to reduce healthcare costs by monitoring and controlling the services provided.
- **Weaknesses**: May limit patients' choice of providers; may prioritize cost-saving over quality.
- **Influence on Nursing**: Care coordination becomes paramount; nurses need to be adept at case management.
- **Role of Nurse Executives**: Oversee contracts, understand stipulations, and ensure the nursing team is aligned with MCO requirements.

**3. Patient-Centered Medical Homes (PCMH):**
- **Strengths**: Focuses on holistic, patient-centered care; interdisciplinary collaboration.
- **Weaknesses**: Implementation barriers, including resistance to change and financial constraints.
- **Influence on Nursing**: Nurses often act as care coordinators, working closely with other healthcare providers.
- **Role of Nurse Executives**: Foster an environment of teamwork, continuous training, and patient-focused care strategies.

**4. Accountable Care Organizations (ACOs):**
- **Strengths**: Focus on quality over quantity; financial incentives for reducing costs and meeting quality benchmarks.
- **Weaknesses**: Complexity in managing contracts and ensuring all providers meet stipulated benchmarks.
- **Influence on Nursing**: Emphasis on evidence-based practice, quality improvement, and interdisciplinary collaboration.
- **Role of Nurse Executives**: Understand the intricacies of ACO contracts, guide quality initiatives, and ensure alignment with ACO goals.

**5. Value-Based Care (VBC):**
- **Strengths**: Payments based on the quality, rather than the quantity, of care.

- **Weaknesses**: Requires robust data analytics; potential financial risks.
- **Influence on Nursing**: Increased focus on preventive care, patient education, and follow-up.
- **Role of Nurse Executives**: Drive quality initiatives, ensure accurate reporting, and foster a culture of excellence.

## 6. Capitation:
- **Strengths**: Providers receive a set amount per patient, regardless of services rendered, encouraging efficiency.
- **Weaknesses**: Can lead to under-utilization of services.
- **Influence on Nursing**: Focus on effective, efficient care; potential for more group-based interventions.
- **Role of Nurse Executives**: Monitor service utilization to ensure neither overuse nor underuse, and manage resources effectively.

## Influences on Care Coordination and Patient Experience:
- **Care Coordination**: Models like PCMH and ACOs emphasize a coordinated approach. This demands that nurses not only provide direct care but also ensure that care is streamlined across the healthcare continuum.
- **Patient Experience**: VBC and PCMH prioritize patient outcomes and satisfaction, driving nursing interventions that are attuned to patient needs, preferences, and feedback.

## Nurse Executives in Navigating Healthcare Models:
Nurse executives act as the keel of the ship, ensuring stability and direction. They must:
- **Understand** each model's intricacies and financial implications.
- **Educate** their teams on the nuances and expectations of each model.
- **Advocate** for resources, training, and tools that enable optimal patient care within each model's framework.
- **Analyze** data and trends to foresee challenges and harness opportunities.
- **Collaborate** with interdisciplinary teams, ensuring that nursing's voice is influential in decision-making processes.

In essence, the healthcare landscape's dynamism is mirrored in its delivery models. For nurse executives, the challenge is not just in understanding these models but in skillfully navigating them to ensure that patient care remains paramount.

# Business Skills:

**Strategic Management in Healthcare**:

**Core Principles and Methodologies:** Strategic management in healthcare revolves around systematic planning and decision-making to achieve long-term objectives and adapt to a constantly evolving environment. At its core, it's a dynamic process that integrates the mission, vision, and values of an organization to set achievable goals.

1. **Environmental Scanning**: This is the process of continually acquiring information on events occurring outside the organization to identify and interpret potential trends. For healthcare settings, this involves monitoring external factors like regulatory changes, technological advancements, socio-economic shifts, and competitive actions. By doing

so, nurse executives can anticipate challenges and opportunities, making the organization proactive rather than reactive.

2. **Goal Setting**: Once potential trends are identified, the next step is to establish clear, measurable, and time-bound objectives. For nurse executives, these goals should align with both patient care outcomes and broader organizational aims. Goals provide direction and a sense of purpose, ensuring everyone is moving cohesively toward the desired future state.

3. **Stakeholder Analysis**: Recognizing and understanding the needs, expectations, and potential influence of various stakeholders is crucial. Stakeholders in healthcare might include patients, families, staff, regulatory bodies, insurers, and even the broader community. By understanding their interests and potential impacts, nurse executives can better address concerns and leverage support.

**Influences on Decision-Making**: These strategic management elements heavily influence decision-making in several ways:

- **Anticipating Change**: With continuous environmental scanning, nurse executives can foresee potential changes in the healthcare landscape, allowing them to pivot strategies or prepare the organization for impending shifts.
- **Aligning Efforts**: Clear goal setting ensures that departmental and individual objectives align with the overall strategy of the healthcare institution. This alignment streamlines efforts, reduces redundancy, and ensures resources are utilized effectively.
- **Balancing Interests**: Stakeholder analysis ensures decisions are balanced, considering the needs and expectations of those most impacted. It promotes a patient-centered approach while also considering the needs of staff and external entities.

**Ensuring Effective Planning and Implementation**:

To ensure the effectiveness of strategic initiatives:

1. **Collaboration is Key**: Nurse executives should foster a culture of collaboration. This involves including multidisciplinary teams in the planning process to garner diverse insights and ensure buy-in.

2. **Continual Monitoring and Feedback**: Strategies should be regularly reviewed against performance metrics. Feedback mechanisms should be in place to understand what's working and what's not, allowing for timely adjustments.

3. **Communication**: Clear communication of the strategic vision, goals, and progress is essential. All members of the healthcare setting should understand their role in achieving the strategy.

4. **Resource Allocation**: Ensure necessary resources (like time, funds, and training) are available to execute the strategy. This might involve reallocating resources based on changing priorities.

In conclusion, strategic management in healthcare is an ongoing process that requires vigilance, adaptability, and collaboration. For nurse executives, leveraging these core principles ensures that the organization remains patient-centered, efficient, and prepared for future challenges and opportunities.

**Evaluation, Feedback, and Continuous Improvement:**

**Techniques and Tools for Evaluation**: In healthcare, the evaluation phase is quintessential. Here are some of the frequently employed techniques:

1. **Key Performance Indicators (KPIs)**: These are measurable values that demonstrate how effectively an organization is achieving key objectives. In a healthcare setting, KPIs might encompass patient satisfaction scores, hospital readmission rates, or infection control rates.
2. **Balanced Scorecard**: This tool provides a balanced view of organizational performance by looking at finances, internal processes, learning/growth, and customer perspectives. For a nursing department, this might mean evaluating financial efficiency, patient care protocols, staff training programs, and patient feedback.
3. **SWOT Analysis**: This assesses strengths, weaknesses, opportunities, and threats. Nurse executives might use this to understand internal capabilities and external challenges.

**Gathering and Interpreting Feedback**: Feedback is the compass that guides adjustments. Here's how nurse executives should approach it:

1. **Staff Feedback**: Regular team meetings, one-on-one sessions, and anonymous suggestion boxes can be effective. Also, employing tools like the Nurse-Family Work Environment Scale can provide insights into the nursing work environment.
2. **Patient Feedback**: Patient satisfaction surveys, like the Hospital Consumer Assessment of Healthcare Providers and Systems (HCAHPS), are invaluable. These standardized surveys capture patients' perspectives on care received.
3. **Other Stakeholders**: Engaging with interdisciplinary teams, attending hospital committee meetings, or collaborating with community partners can provide broader feedback.

Interpreting this feedback requires a mix of data analytics and empathy. Quantitative data from surveys provides a numerical assessment, while qualitative feedback (like comments or interviews) offers a deeper understanding of underlying issues or positive outcomes.

**Continuous Improvement Practices**: Post-evaluation, the journey doesn't end. Continuous improvement ensures that healthcare settings adapt and evolve:

1. **Plan-Do-Check-Act (PDCA)**: A cyclic methodology used to achieve continuous improvement. Start with planning (design or revise processes), then do (implement the plan), check (assess the results), and finally act (adjust and refine the processes).
2. **Lean and Six Sigma**: These methodologies focus on reducing waste and variability in processes. In healthcare, they can optimize patient flows, reduce medication errors, and improve overall care quality.
3. **Benchmarking**: Comparing your organization's processes and performance metrics to industry bests or best practices from other institutions. It helps identify areas of improvement and potential strategies.

For nurse executives, the cycle of planning, execution, evaluation, feedback, and improvement is ceaseless. It's not just about meeting benchmarks, but consistently raising the bar. For instance, if patient feedback indicates dissatisfaction with waiting times, continuous improvement might involve streamlining admission procedures or enhancing staff training.

In essence, the success of healthcare delivery hinges on the ability to evaluate current practices accurately, embrace feedback, and instill a culture of continuous refinement. For nurse executives, mastering these elements not only leads to better patient outcomes but also fosters a work environment where excellence is the norm, not the exception.

**Risk Management for Nurse Executives**:

**The Imperative of Risk Management**: Risk management in nursing leadership is not just about minimizing liabilities but also about ensuring patient safety, maintaining quality care, and preserving the organization's reputation. In the rapidly evolving healthcare landscape, potential risks—from patient care errors to regulatory non-compliance—can have profound implications. For nurse executives, proactively managing these risks is paramount to fostering trust among patients, staff, and other stakeholders.

**Systematic Process of Risk Management**:

1. **Identification**: The first step is recognizing potential risks. This could be through incident reports, patient complaints, staff feedback, or data analytics. Regular audits, both internal and external, can help spot potential risk areas.
2. **Assessment**: Once identified, risks need to be assessed based on their potential impact and likelihood of occurrence. Tools such as risk matrices or risk heat maps can be used. For instance, a medication error due to a system flaw would be assessed as a high-impact and high-likelihood risk, necessitating immediate attention.
3. **Prioritization**: Not all risks carry equal weight. Nurse executives must prioritize risks to ensure that resources are allocated effectively. High-impact, high-likelihood risks are typically addressed first, while lower-tier risks might be monitored or accepted.

**Top Mitigation Strategies**:

1. **Clinical Risk Management**:
   - **Evidence-Based Practice**: Adhering to the latest evidence-based guidelines ensures that patients receive the best possible care, minimizing the potential for errors.
   - **Continuing Education**: Regular training for the nursing staff on emerging care practices, technology usage, and regulatory changes is essential.
   - **Clinical Protocols and Checklists**: These can be invaluable in standardizing care processes, ensuring that no step is overlooked.
   - **Effective Communication**: Many clinical errors stem from miscommunication. Implementing tools like SBAR (Situation, Background, Assessment, Recommendation) can streamline clinical communication.
2. **Operational Risk Management**:
   - **Regulatory Compliance**: Staying updated with local, state, and federal regulations is vital. Regular compliance training and audits can prevent potential legal entanglements.
   - **Technology and System Upgrades**: Keeping abreast of the latest healthcare technologies can reduce operational inefficiencies. For example, implementing a

state-of-the-art Electronic Health Record (EHR) system can reduce documentation errors.
- **Incident Reporting Systems**: These allow for real-time reporting of any mishaps, ensuring quick resolution and providing data for future preventive measures.
- **Crisis Management Plans**: Having a well-defined plan for crises, be it a public health emergency or a data breach, ensures that the organization can respond swiftly and effectively.

Risk management is a dynamic and ongoing process. For nurse executives, it's about striking the right balance between being proactive in identifying and mitigating risks and being responsive when unforeseen challenges arise. Ultimately, effective risk management not only shields the organization but also ensures that patients receive safe, high-quality care.

**Financial Management Essentials for Nurse Executives**:

**Fundamentals of Financial Management**: Healthcare financial management intertwines clinical practice with economic principles. While patient care remains the prime directive, understanding and managing the finances ensure sustainability and quality of service.

1. **Budgeting**: A budget serves as a financial roadmap, detailing where resources come from and how they will be spent. For nurse executives, budgeting requires:
   - **Direct Costs**: These are directly tied to patient care, such as salaries of nurses, medications, and medical supplies.
   - **Indirect Costs**: These might include utilities, administrative salaries, and facility maintenance.
   - **Capital Expenditures**: These are significant, one-time expenses like purchasing new equipment or facility renovations.
2. **Forecasting**: This is the art and science of predicting future financial trends based on historical data and current market conditions. Forecasting allows nurse executives to anticipate changes in patient volume, funding sources, or care costs, and adjust strategies accordingly.
3. **Financial Statements**: These documents give an overview of an organization's financial health.
   - **Income Statement**: Shows revenues, expenses, and profits over a specific period.
   - **Balance Sheet**: Provides a snapshot of assets, liabilities, and equity at a particular point in time.
   - **Cash Flow Statement**: Chronicles the inflow and outflow of cash, indicating how an organization manages its liquid assets.

**Leveraging Financial Insights**:

1. **Clinical Excellence**: By understanding the financial elements, nurse executives can identify high-cost areas and seek out best practices to improve efficiency without compromising care. For instance, if a particular unit has unusually high overtime costs, a deeper dive might reveal scheduling inefficiencies or understaffing, leading to corrective actions.

2. **Administrative Excellence**: Financial insights allow nurse executives to:
   - Optimize resource allocation: ensuring departments are adequately funded and staffed.
   - Make informed decisions on purchases: evaluating the ROI of new technologies or equipment.
   - Manage financial relationships: understanding contracts, reimbursements, and negotiations with suppliers or insurance providers.
3. **Strategic Initiatives**: Beyond daily operations, financial knowledge aids nurse executives in strategic planning. Whether considering a new wing, launching a community outreach program, or upgrading IT systems, understanding the financial implications is crucial.
4. **Stakeholder Communication**: Nurse executives often liaise with hospital boards, investors, and other stakeholders. Being fluent in financial language strengthens these communications, ensuring stakeholders are informed and confident in the organization's direction.

**Practical Application**: Imagine a nurse executive is considering introducing a new telehealth service. By analyzing forecasted data, they can project potential patient demand, technology costs, and staffing needs. They would examine budget constraints to ensure affordability and study financial statements to gauge the financial health of the organization. If, for instance, the cash flow statement indicates tight liquidity, the executive might seek external funding or phase the rollout to manage costs.

In sum, while financial management might seem a departure from the clinical aspects of a nurse executive's role, it's undeniably integral. By mastering these financial essentials, nurse executives ensure that their organizations remain financially viable, adaptive, and primed to offer the best patient care possible.

# EXAM PREP SECTION:

Welcome to the practice test section of your ANCC Nurse Executive exam preparation guide. Here, you'll have an opportunity to test your knowledge and assess your readiness for the actual exam.

We understand the importance of not just knowing the answer, but understanding the reasoning behind it. That's why, uniquely, we've designed this section to provide the answer and its comprehensive explanation immediately following each question. This immediate feedback approach is grounded in educational psychology principles, aiding in the reinforcement of knowledge and immediate correction of misconceptions. It minimizes the chances of repeated mistakes, accelerates your learning curve, and ensures a more productive and efficient study session. So make sure you take out a peice of paper or something to hide the answer and prevent peaking and seeing the answer.

Dive in, challenge yourself, and remember: every mistake is a learning opportunity. Let's begin.

1. A nurse executive is reviewing the hospital's financial statements. Which of the following would be directly impacted by a department's consistent under-staffing?
A) Gross Margin
B) Operating Income
C) Total Equity
D) Fixed Assets

Answer: B) Operating Income. Explanation: Under-staffing can lead to inefficiencies and increased overtime costs, which would directly affect the hospital's operating income. While other financial metrics might be indirectly influenced, the operating income reflects the core operations of the hospital, including staffing.

2. A local community hospital is looking to expand its services to include a new oncology department. As a nurse executive, which of the following should be your FIRST step?
A) Hiring oncology specialists
B) Purchasing oncology equipment
C) Conducting a community needs assessment
D) Launching an advertising campaign for the new department

Answer: C) Conducting a community needs assessment. Explanation: Before expanding services or investing in resources, it's essential to determine if there's a genuine need within the community. A community needs assessment will provide data on the demand for oncology services, helping to guide subsequent decisions.

3. A patient has voiced concerns about their privacy rights being violated during their hospital stay. As a nurse executive, you are aware that which act provides the primary guidelines for patient health information privacy?
A) ADA (Americans with Disabilities Act)
B) HIPAA (Health Insurance Portability and Accountability Act)
C) FMLA (Family and Medical Leave Act)
D) EMTALA (Emergency Medical Treatment & Labor Act)

Answer: B) HIPAA (Health Insurance Portability and Accountability Act). Explanation: HIPAA provides the national standards for protecting the privacy of individual health information. Any concerns about patient privacy rights in a healthcare setting would primarily be addressed under HIPAA guidelines.

4. You are a nurse executive at a teaching hospital. Which of the following strategies would be LEAST effective in promoting a culture of continuous improvement?
A) Encouraging staff to report errors without fear of retribution
B) Implementing evidence-based practices in patient care
C) Conducting yearly performance reviews without feedback sessions
D) Establishing inter-departmental collaboration for best practice sharing

Answer: C) Conducting yearly performance reviews without feedback sessions Explanation: Continuous improvement is fostered by ongoing feedback and open communication. Conducting performance reviews without feedback sessions misses an opportunity for growth, reflection, and improvement.

5. A nurse executive is working to enhance the organizational structure of a healthcare facility. Recognizing the various types of structures, which design emphasizes a more decentralized decision-making process, emphasizing departmental specialization?
a. Matrix structure
b. Flat structure
c. Functional structure
d. Divisional structure

Answer: c. Functional structure
Explanation: A functional organizational structure divides the organization based on specialized functional areas such as IT, finance, or nursing. This decentralizes decision-making as decisions tend to be made within specific functional departments.

6. In the midst of a significant organizational change, a nurse executive recognizes the importance of acknowledging and navigating the informal organizational structure. Why is this considered vital?
a. It involves top-tier management only.
b. It underscores the written policies of the institution.
c. It captures the essence of how work truly gets done.
d. It primarily revolves around the facility's budget.

Answer: c. It captures the essence of how work truly gets done.
Explanation: The informal organizational structure refers to interrelationships within an organization that aren't outlined in official documents. It includes the unwritten, social aspects of organizational life which often reflect the actual interactions and power dynamics.

7. A nurse executive wants to implement a new electronic health record (EHR) system. Which structural element should the executive primarily focus on to ensure that nurses can seamlessly adopt the new EHR across the facility?
a. Organizational hierarchy
b. Workflow processes
c. Departmental divisions
d. Corporate branding

Answer: b. Workflow processes
Explanation: Ensuring that the EHR aligns with and enhances existing workflow processes will help in its adoption. Adjustments might be needed to workflows, but understanding the current process is essential.

8. When evaluating the organizational environment, a nurse executive identifies certain informal leaders who influence their peers despite not having formal leadership titles. These leaders are termed as:
a. Proxies
b. Champions
c. Delegates
d. Mavericks

Answer: b. Champions
Explanation: Informal leaders who are positive and influential, promoting and championing new ideas or changes within an organization, are often referred to as champions.

9. An organization is designed in such a way that teams are formed based on products, with each product type having its team which includes members from various functional areas. This type of organizational design is called:
a. Functional structure
b. Matrix structure
c. Hierarchical structure
d. Product-based divisional structure

Answer: d. Product-based divisional structure
Explanation: In a product-based divisional structure, divisions are created based on the type of product. Each division then contains all the necessary resources and functions within it.

10. During an organizational restructuring, a nurse executive is considering the span of control for nursing managers. A wider span of control would:
a. Increase the levels of hierarchy in the organization.
b. Reduce the direct reports a manager has.
c. Decrease the overall efficiency of the organization.
d. Allow a manager to oversee more direct reports.

Answer: d. Allow a manager to oversee more direct reports.
Explanation: The span of control refers to the number of subordinates a manager can efficiently and effectively manage. A wider span means more direct reports per manager.

11. Recognizing the significance of external environmental factors, a nurse executive is particularly focused on potential legislative changes. This is a prime example of the:
a. Socio-cultural environment.
b. Task environment.
c. Macro-environment.
d. Internal environment.

Answer: c. Macro-environment.
Explanation: The macro-environment includes the larger societal forces that affect the whole micro-environment, such as legislative changes, economic conditions, and technological shifts.

12. A nurse executive, when analyzing the organizational environment, acknowledges the critical role of certain organizations directly linked and regularly interacting with the healthcare facility. These organizations form part of the:
a. Internal environment.
b. Competitive environment.
c. Task environment.
d. Cultural environment.

Answer: c. Task environment.
Explanation: The task environment includes entities that directly affect an organization and have a vested interest in its performance, such as suppliers, competitors, and regulatory agencies.

13. The healthcare facility is transitioning to a model where the decision-making process involves employees at all levels, fostering a sense of ownership and participation. This model is best described as:
a. Centralized decision-making
b. Hierarchical structure
c. Decentralized decision-making
d. Linear structure

Answer: c. Decentralized decision-making
Explanation: Decentralized decision-making allows for decision-making processes to occur at various levels in the organization, promoting broader involvement and often faster responses to challenges.

14. For effective organizational management, a nurse executive emphasizes the alignment of the hospital's strategies, goals, and values. This ensures that:
a. The facility can accommodate more patients.
b. There's reduced emphasis on quality care.
c. Resources are aligned to achieve strategic goals.
d. Immediate financial gains are realized.

Answer: c. Resources are aligned to achieve strategic goals.
Explanation: Ensuring alignment between strategies, goals, and values guarantees that everyone is moving in the same direction and resources are utilized efficiently toward achieving the organization's objectives.

15. In the healthcare organization's board of directors, who is typically responsible for ensuring clinical quality across the organization?
a. Chief Financial Officer
b. Chief Executive Officer
c. Chief Nursing Officer
d. Chief Marketing Officer


Answer: c. Chief Nursing Officer
Explanation: Within healthcare organizations, the Chief Nursing Officer (CNO) often plays a critical role in overseeing clinical quality, patient care standards, and nursing practice across the organization.

16. Which governance model emphasizes a collaborative approach between clinicians and administrators to ensure high-quality care?
a. Shareholder Model
b. Stakeholder Model
c. Clinical Integration Model
d. Corporate Model



Answer: c. Clinical Integration Model
Explanation: The Clinical Integration Model focuses on inter-professional collaboration, ensuring that both clinical and administrative perspectives are considered in decision-making processes related to patient care and quality.

17. A healthcare organization is considering expanding its services. Who among the following would typically be MOST involved in assessing the feasibility and implications of this expansion?
a. Director of Nursing
b. Governance Board
c. Frontline Clinical Staff
d. Patient Advocacy Group



Answer: b. Governance Board
Explanation: The governance board is responsible for making high-level strategic decisions for the organization, which includes decisions about expansion, allocation of resources, and ensuring alignment with the organization's mission.

18. Which of the following best describes the fiduciary duty of a healthcare organization's board of directors?
a. Guaranteeing profits to shareholders
b. Actively managing day-to-day operations
c. Ensuring ethical and financial integrity in decision-making
d. Organizing community health fairs

Answer: c. Ensuring ethical and financial integrity in decision-making
Explanation: The board's fiduciary duty is to act in the best interest of the organization, which encompasses ensuring ethical and financial integrity.

19. Which aspect of governance is concerned with how decisions are made and who makes them within the healthcare organization?
a. Financial Oversight
b. Decision-making Authority
c. Stakeholder Representation
d. Clinical Quality Assurance

Answer: b. Decision-making Authority
Explanation: Decision-making authority relates directly to the process, hierarchy, and delegation of decision-making within an organization.

20. In a healthcare organization that adopts the Carver Model of governance, what is the board's primary focus?
a. Operational management
b. Outcomes and organizational ends
c. Clinical procedures
d. Fundraising

Answer: b. Outcomes and organizational ends. Explanation: The Carver Model emphasizes a focus on the outcomes and the ends, meaning the board concentrates on the organization's broader goals and leaves operational matters to executives.

21. Which of the following is NOT typically a responsibility of a healthcare organization's governance board?
a. Hiring and evaluating the CEO
b. Direct patient care
c. Setting strategic direction
d. Ensuring financial viability

Answer: b. Direct patient care
Explanation: The governance board is focused on high-level organizational oversight, not direct patient care, which is the responsibility of clinical staff.

22. In terms of governance, what is the primary purpose of a board's finance committee in a healthcare organization?
a. Recruiting clinicians
b. Overseeing financial policies and performance
c. Directly managing financial transactions
d. Setting clinical quality standards

Answer: b. Overseeing financial policies and performance
Explanation: A board's finance committee is tasked with monitoring the organization's financial health, ensuring adherence to financial policies, and guiding financial decisions.

23. To whom does the Chief Executive Officer (CEO) of a healthcare organization typically report directly?
a. Chief Medical Officer
b. The organization's shareholders
c. The governance board
d. The patient advisory committee

Answer: c. The governance board
Explanation: In most healthcare organizations, the CEO is accountable to the governance board, which provides oversight and direction.

24. In the context of healthcare governance, what is the primary focus of the "triple aim"?
a. Finance, operations, and marketing
b. Patient care, staff satisfaction, and community outreach
c. Patient experience, health of populations, and per capita cost
d. Clinical outcomes, patient throughput, and profitability

Answer: c. Patient experience, health of populations, and per capita cost
Explanation: The "triple aim," introduced by the Institute for Healthcare Improvement, focuses on enhancing the patient experience, improving the health of populations, and reducing the per capita cost of healthcare.

25. In a typical healthcare organization, who is directly responsible for the overall operational and strategic management?
a. Chief Medical Officer
b. Chief Nursing Executive
c. Board Chairperson
d. Chief Executive Officer

Answer: d. Chief Executive Officer
Explanation: The CEO has overarching responsibility for both strategic direction and operational management of a healthcare organization.

26. The role of which individual primarily focuses on the medical oversight, quality assurance, and leadership of the physician team?
a. Director of Nursing
b. Chief Financial Officer
c. Chief Medical Officer
d. Governance Board Chair

Answer: c. Chief Medical Officer
Explanation: The Chief Medical Officer provides leadership to the physician team and oversees clinical quality and safety.

27. In a healthcare organization's governance structure, who typically plays a critical role in bridging the gap between clinical staff and executive leadership?
a. Chief Human Resources Officer
b. Chief Nursing Officer
c. Chief Information Officer
d. Chief Executive Officer

Answer: b. Chief Nursing Officer
Explanation: The Chief Nursing Officer represents the nursing staff at the executive level, ensuring that clinical perspectives are included in decision-making processes.

28. The primary role of which individual is to ensure the financial viability and sustainability of the healthcare organization?
a. Chief Financial Officer
b. Chief Medical Officer
c. Governance Board Chair
d. Director of Marketing

Answer: a. Chief Financial Officer
Explanation: The CFO oversees financial management, ensuring that the organization remains financially viable and sustainable.

29. In governance, whose primary responsibility is to ensure that the voice of the patients and community is represented in the healthcare organization's decisions?
a. Director of Community Relations
b. Patient Advocate
c. Chief Operating Officer
d. Chief Quality Officer

Answer: b. Patient Advocate
Explanation: The Patient Advocate's role is to ensure that patient concerns, feedback, and rights are represented and addressed at the organizational level.

30. Which role is primarily responsible for overseeing the technological infrastructure of the healthcare organization and ensuring the integration of IT solutions to improve patient care?
a. Chief Information Officer
b. Chief Quality Officer
c. Chief Medical Officer
d. Director of Nursing

Answer: a. Chief Information Officer
Explanation: The CIO oversees the technological aspects of the organization, ensuring that IT solutions align with the goals of improving patient care and operational efficiency.

31. Who typically oversees the quality and safety of patient care, ensuring that standards are met and continually improved upon?
a. Chief Executive Officer
b. Chief Operations Officer
c. Chief Medical Officer
d. Chief Quality Officer

Answer: d. Chief Quality Officer
Explanation: The Chief Quality Officer's primary focus is on ensuring and enhancing the quality and safety of patient care through standards, policies, and continuous improvement initiatives.

32. In terms of governance, which role is primarily responsible for the day-to-day operations and management of the healthcare facility?
a. Chief Financial Officer
b. Chief Operating Officer
c. Chief Medical Officer
d. Director of Community Outreach

Answer: b. Chief Operating Officer. Explanation: The COO is typically in charge of day-to-day operations, ensuring that the healthcare facility runs smoothly and efficiently.

33. Which individual plays a critical role in attracting, retaining, and managing the workforce of the healthcare organization?
a. Chief Human Resources Officer
b. Chief Medical Officer
c. Director of Nursing
d. Chief Financial Officer

Answer: a. Chief Human Resources Officer. Explanation: The Chief Human Resources Officer oversees all aspects of workforce management, including recruitment, retention, and employee relations.

34. Whose main responsibility in a healthcare governance structure is to lead and guide the board, ensuring effective governance processes and adherence to the organization's mission and vision?
a. Chief Executive Officer
b. Chief Medical Officer
c. Board Chairperson
d. Chief Nursing Officer

Answer: c. Board Chairperson. Explanation: The Board Chairperson leads and guides the governance board, ensuring alignment with the organization's mission, vision, and governance processes.

35. Which governance structure primarily relies on a single board that oversees both the strategic and operational aspects of a healthcare organization?
a. Unitary Board
b. Two-Tier Board
c. Advisory Board
d. Functional Board

Answer: a. Unitary Board
Explanation: A Unitary Board is a single-tiered board where both the executive and non-executive directors sit together, overseeing both the strategic and operational functions of the organization.

36. In a healthcare system with multiple hospitals and facilities, which governance structure often has a central governing body that provides broad oversight while each facility may have its own local board?
a. Centralized Governance
b. Federated Governance
c. Matrix Governance
d. Collaborative Governance

Answer: b. Federated Governance
Explanation: In a Federated Governance structure, a central governing body provides overarching governance while individual facilities or hospitals may have local boards responsible for local issues.

37. Which governance structure is characterized by a clear separation between the management board, which oversees day-to-day operations, and a supervisory board, which focuses on strategic oversight?
a. Unitary Board
b. Two-Tier Board
c. Matrix Governance
d. Centralized Governance

Answer: b. Two-Tier Board
Explanation: In a Two-Tier Board, there is a clear distinction between the management board responsible for daily operations and a supervisory board responsible for broader strategic oversight.

38. Which governance structure involves collaboration between multiple entities or stakeholders, with each having shared accountability and decision-making responsibilities?
a. Matrix Governance
b. Collaborative Governance
c. Centralized Governance
d. Unitary Board

Answer: b. Collaborative Governance
Explanation: Collaborative Governance involves shared governance among multiple stakeholders, emphasizing collaboration, shared decision-making, and mutual accountability.

39. In which governance structure does a healthcare organization rely heavily on committees or teams organized around specific functions, such as quality or finance?
a. Matrix Governance
b. Functional Governance
c. Federated Governance
d. Collaborative Governance

Answer: b. Functional Governance
Explanation: Functional Governance relies on committees or teams organized around specific operational or clinical functions, ensuring specialized focus on key areas.

40. Which governance structure is characterized by vertical and horizontal reporting relationships, often used in complex organizations to balance functional and product lines?
a. Centralized Governance
b. Two-Tier Board
c. Matrix Governance
d. Functional Governance

Answer: c. Matrix Governance
Explanation: Matrix Governance involves both vertical (hierarchical) and horizontal (functional or product line) reporting relationships, ensuring flexibility and adaptability in complex organizations.

41. In which governance model is decision-making primarily centralized at the top level, with lower levels mainly executing those decisions?
a. Centralized Governance
b. Collaborative Governance
c. Federated Governance
d. Matrix Governance

Answer: a. Centralized Governance
Explanation: In Centralized Governance, decision-making authority is primarily held at the top, with lower organizational levels executing those decisions.

42. Which governance structure primarily serves to offer non-binding strategic advice to the organization, often without formal decision-making authority?
a. Advisory Board
b. Unitary Board
c. Functional Board
d. Collaborative Board

Answer: a. Advisory Board. Explanation: Advisory Boards offer strategic advice and insights without having formal authority or decision-making responsibilities in the organization.

43. In a healthcare organization that emphasizes a shared governance model, who typically has a significant role in decision-making processes, especially concerning clinical practices?
a. External Consultants
b. Administrative Executives
c. Clinical Staff and Nurses
d. Financial Analysts

Answer: c. Clinical Staff and Nurses
Explanation: Shared governance models emphasize the active participation of clinical staff, including nurses, in decision-making processes related to clinical practices and patient care.

44. Which governance structure is characterized by a focus on stakeholder engagement, often involving external community members in decision-making processes?
a. Community Governance
b. Matrix Governance
c. Centralized Governance
d. Functional Governance

Answer: a. Community Governance. Explanation: Community Governance places a strong emphasis on involving external community members and stakeholders in the governance and decision-making processes, ensuring the organization's alignment with community needs and values.

45. Which governance mechanism involves regular and systematic assessment of an organization's performance against pre-established criteria or benchmarks?
a. Performance Appraisal
b. Stakeholder Engagement
c. Quality Audits
d. Balanced Scorecard

Answer: c. Quality Audits
Explanation: Quality Audits involve the systematic evaluation of an organization's performance against specific standards or benchmarks to ensure quality and compliance.

46. Within the context of governance, what is the primary purpose of a mechanism like the "Balanced Scorecard"?
a. To assess financial viability only.
b. To solely gauge patient satisfaction metrics.
c. To ensure clinical staff competency through rigorous assessment.
d. To provide a holistic view of an organization's performance across multiple domains.

Answer: d. To provide a holistic view of an organization's performance across multiple domains.
Explanation: The Balanced Scorecard offers a comprehensive overview of an organization's performance, including financial, customer, internal process, and learning and growth perspectives.

47. Which governance mechanism seeks to involve individuals, groups, or organizations that may be affected by or can affect the outcomes of a decision?
a. Performance Appraisal
b. Stakeholder Engagement
c. Quality Audits
d. Risk Management

Answer: b. Stakeholder Engagement
Explanation: Stakeholder Engagement is the process of involving all relevant parties in decision-making processes, ensuring their perspectives and interests are considered.

48. A key mechanism in governance that systematically addresses potential threats and opportunities to ensure organizational objectives are met is known as:
a. SWOT Analysis
b. Risk Management
c. Financial Forecasting
d. Performance Benchmarking

Answer: b. Risk Management
Explanation: Risk Management involves identifying, assessing, and prioritizing potential threats and opportunities to ensure that organizational goals are achieved with minimized disruptions.

49. Which governance mechanism primarily focuses on aligning individual performance with organizational goals and providing feedback for professional development?
a. Performance Appraisal
b. Stakeholder Analysis
c. Risk Analysis
d. Financial Forecasting

Answer: a. Performance Appraisal
Explanation: Performance Appraisal is the process of evaluating and providing feedback on an individual's performance in alignment with organizational objectives.

50. In governance structures, which mechanism involves regularly checking and verifying the financial records of an organization to ensure accuracy and compliance?
a. Financial Analysis
b. Financial Audit
c. Budget Forecast
d. SWOT Analysis

Answer: b. Financial Audit. Explanation: A Financial Audit is a comprehensive examination of an organization's financial records to ensure accuracy, transparency, and compliance with accounting standards and regulations.

51. Which governance mechanism provides a structured process to identify strengths, weaknesses, opportunities, and threats for strategic planning?
a. Risk Management
b. Performance Appraisal
c. Financial Forecasting
d. SWOT Analysis

Answer: d. SWOT Analysis. Explanation: SWOT Analysis is a strategic planning tool used to identify and evaluate the Strengths, Weaknesses, Opportunities, and Threats related to business competition or project planning.

52. What governance mechanism involves projecting future financial trends based on past and present financial data?
a. Financial Audit
b. Financial Analysis
c. Financial Forecasting
d. Risk Assessment

Answer: c. Financial Forecasting
Explanation: Financial Forecasting involves predicting future financial outcomes by analyzing and interpreting past and present financial data.

53. For healthcare organizations, which governance mechanism focuses on preventing, detecting, and responding to infections, ensuring the safety and health of patients and staff?
a. Risk Management
b. Infection Control
c. Stakeholder Engagement
d. SWOT Analysis

Answer: b. Infection Control
Explanation: Infection Control involves implementing measures and protocols to prevent the spread of infections within healthcare settings, ensuring patient and staff safety.

54. In governance, which mechanism is employed to ensure that policies and procedures of a healthcare organization align with external regulations and standards?
a. Policy Review and Alignment
b. Risk Assessment
c. Financial Benchmarking
d. Performance Appraisal

Answer: a. Policy Review and Alignment
Explanation: Policy Review and Alignment ensures that the internal policies and procedures of an organization are in compliance with external regulations and standards, ensuring both efficacy and compliance.

55. In the context of healthcare, which of the following best describes the role of organizational culture?
a. The written policies and procedures that dictate behavior.
b. The tangible assets such as equipment and infrastructure.
c. The shared values, beliefs, and practices that shape behavior and decision-making.
d. The regular financial audits and checks.

Answer: c. The shared values, beliefs, and practices that shape behavior and decision-making.
Explanation: Organizational culture refers to the intangible shared values, beliefs, and practices within an organization that influence behaviors and decisions.

56. How does a strong organizational culture impact patient care in a healthcare setting?
a. It reduces the need for equipment and resources.
b. It ensures financial success without regard to patient outcomes.
c. It leads to consistent practices and behaviors that align with organizational values.
d. It minimizes the need for governance structures.

Answer: c. It leads to consistent practices and behaviors that align with organizational values.
Explanation: A strong organizational culture promotes consistency in practices and behaviors, which, when aligned with organizational values, ensures better patient care.

57. Which of the following is true about the relationship between governance and organizational culture in a healthcare setting?
a. Governance structures replace the need for a strong organizational culture.
b. Governance structures and organizational culture operate in isolation.
c. Governance structures can help reinforce and shape organizational culture.
d. Organizational culture solely dictates the governance structures.

Answer: c. Governance structures can help reinforce and shape organizational culture.
Explanation: Governance structures provide the framework, while organizational culture fills that framework with shared values, beliefs, and practices.

58. Which of the following is a potential consequence of a misalignment between governance and organizational culture in healthcare?
a. Seamless communication and decision-making processes.
b. Enhanced patient satisfaction scores.
c. Conflicts, decreased morale, and potential reductions in patient care quality.
d. Increased financial profitability.

Answer: c. Conflicts, decreased morale, and potential reductions in patient care quality.
Explanation: A misalignment can result in conflicts and inconsistencies in practices, which can adversely affect morale and patient care.

59. How can organizational culture influence the decision-making process in healthcare?
a. By dictating the financial investments of the organization.
b. By shaping the perceptions, attitudes, and values that guide decisions.
c. By determining the physical infrastructure of the healthcare facility.
d. By setting fixed rules for every decision.

Answer: b. By shaping the perceptions, attitudes, and values that guide decisions.
Explanation: Organizational culture influences the way members perceive situations, weigh options, and ultimately make decisions.

60. Which of the following best describes how leaders can positively influence organizational culture in healthcare?
a. By enforcing strict rules and policies without exceptions.
b. By modeling desired behaviors, communicating values, and rewarding aligned behaviors.
c. By isolating themselves from daily operations and challenges.
d. By focusing solely on financial outcomes.

Answer: b. By modeling desired behaviors, communicating values, and rewarding aligned behaviors.
Explanation: Leaders play a pivotal role in shaping culture by setting examples, reinforcing values, and recognizing and rewarding behaviors that align with the desired culture.

61. Which element is crucial for embedding a change in organizational culture within a healthcare setting?
a. Implementing a one-time training session.
b. Focusing solely on top management behavior.
c. Consistent reinforcement and alignment of values across all levels.
d. Disregarding feedback from frontline staff.

Answer: c. Consistent reinforcement and alignment of values across all levels.
Explanation: For a cultural change to take root, consistent reinforcement and alignment of values across all organizational levels are essential.

62. In the context of healthcare, why is understanding and assessing organizational culture vital?
a. It helps in determining the market value of the organization.
b. It provides insights into potential areas of conflict, strengths, and areas for improvement.
c. It reduces the need for technological upgrades.
d. It solely determines the compensation packages for employees.

Answer: b. It provides insights into potential areas of conflict, strengths, and areas for improvement.
Explanation: Understanding the organizational culture gives insights into the behavioral dynamics of the organization, helping in identifying potential challenges and leveraging strengths.

63. Which of the following can be a significant barrier to changing organizational culture in a healthcare setting?
a. Strong financial reserves.
b. Resistance from members accustomed to existing culture.
c. Implementation of advanced medical technology.
d. External marketing campaigns.

Answer: b. Resistance from members accustomed to existing culture. Explanation: Change often faces resistance, especially from those accustomed to and comfortable with the existing culture. This resistance can be a significant barrier to cultural transformation.

64. How can governance structures support a desired organizational culture shift in a healthcare organization?
a. By ignoring the current organizational culture completely.
b. By setting policies and practices that align with and reinforce the desired culture.
c. By ensuring that the organization remains static and change-resistant.
d. By focusing only on external stakeholder demands.

Answer: b. By setting policies and practices that align with and reinforce the desired culture. Explanation: Governance structures, through policies and practices, can provide the necessary framework to guide, support, and reinforce the desired shift in organizational culture.

65. As a nurse executive, which of the following would you consider to be the primary driver for promoting safety and excellence in care?
a. Reducing costs associated with patient care.
b. Enhancing the public image and reputation of the institution.
c. Meeting the minimal standards set by regulators.
d. Improving patient outcomes and increasing staff satisfaction.

Answer: d. Improving patient outcomes and increasing staff satisfaction. Explanation: While all options have their importance, the primary driver should always be improving patient outcomes and ensuring the well-being and satisfaction of staff.

66. When considering the introduction of a new clinical protocol, what is the most effective strategy to ensure its successful implementation?
a. Announce the protocol at a staff meeting.
b. Offer financial incentives for its adoption.
c. Involve frontline staff in its development and training.
d. Implement without feedback, relying on its scientific backing.

Answer: c. Involve frontline staff in its development and training.
Explanation: Engaging frontline staff in the development and training ensures that they understand, buy into, and feel a part of the change, which typically leads to better adherence.

67. Which of the following would be an appropriate Key Performance Indicator (KPI) for safety and excellence in a healthcare setting?
a. Number of coffee breaks taken by staff.
b. Patient wait time for elective procedures.
c. Frequency of staff attending outside seminars.
d. Incidence of hospital-acquired infections.

Answer: d. Incidence of hospital-acquired infections.
Explanation: Hospital-acquired infections directly relate to patient safety and care quality. Monitoring and reducing these infections is a prime indicator of promoting safety and excellence.

68. In promoting a culture of safety, a nurse executive should prioritize:
a. Punishing those who make errors to set an example.
b. Encouraging a blame-free reporting environment.
c. Ignoring minor safety breaches to focus on major ones.
d. Focusing solely on patient feedback for safety improvements.

Answer: b. Encouraging a blame-free reporting environment.
Explanation: A blame-free environment encourages staff to report errors and near misses, which can then be addressed and prevented in the future.

69. The use of evidence-based practices in nursing ensures:
a. Reduced need for nurse training.
b. A shift away from patient-centered care.
c. Practices are rooted in research and proven efficacy.
d. Nurses rely more on intuition than evidence.

Answer: c. Practices are rooted in research and proven efficacy.
Explanation: Evidence-based practices are those that have been researched and have demonstrated effectiveness, ensuring care is based on proven strategies.

70. To promote excellence in care, it's crucial for a nurse executive to:
a. Implement policies without staff feedback.
b. Focus solely on the most experienced nurses for insights.
c. Encourage continuous learning and professional development.
d. Rely on outdated but familiar protocols.

Answer: c. Encourage continuous learning and professional development.
Explanation: Excellence is an ongoing pursuit, and by promoting continuous learning and development, a nurse executive ensures that staff are always at the forefront of best practices.

71. Which strategy can be implemented to improve safety in a high-stress environment like an emergency room?
a. Increasing patient wait times to ensure thoroughness.
b. Relying on ad-hoc communication methods during peak times.
c. Implementing standardized checklists for common procedures.
d. Reducing staff during peak hours to decrease chaos.

Answer: c. Implementing standardized checklists for common procedures.
Explanation: Checklists ensure that all steps are followed, particularly in high-stress situations, and can significantly reduce errors.

72. What role does leadership play in promoting safety and excellence in care?
a. Leadership plays a minor role; frontline staff drive safety.
b. Leaders set the tone, model desired behaviors, and create a supportive environment.
c. Leadership should strictly enforce rules without explaining their importance.
d. Leaders should prioritize financial metrics over safety.

Answer: b. Leaders set the tone, model desired behaviors, and create a supportive environment.
Explanation: Effective leadership creates a culture where safety and excellence are prioritized, and everyone feels supported in these goals.

73. For a nurse executive, promoting interprofessional collaboration can lead to:
a. Increased competition among staff members.
b. Siloed departments focusing on individual goals.
c. Enhanced patient care through shared knowledge and expertise.
d. A diminished role for nursing within the healthcare team.

Answer: c. Enhanced patient care through shared knowledge and expertise.
Explanation: Interprofessional collaboration brings together the strengths and expertise of various professionals, leading to more holistic and improved patient care.

74. In ensuring excellence, it's important for nurse executives to:
a. Discourage feedback that may seem critical.
b. Focus solely on positive patient outcomes, ignoring near misses.
c. Regularly review and update protocols based on new evidence and feedback.
d. Stick to traditional practices to maintain consistency.

Answer: c. Regularly review and update protocols based on new evidence and feedback.
Explanation: Excellence requires continuous adaptation and improvement, and updating protocols based on new findings and feedback ensures the highest standard of care is maintained.

75. To successfully change organizational culture, it's essential for a nurse executive to first:
a. Implement changes without any assessment.
b. Understand and identify the existing culture.
c. Establish a strict top-down approach for change.
d. Isolate departments that resist change.

Answer: b. Understand and identify the existing culture.
Explanation: Before initiating change, understanding the current state is crucial. Recognizing the prevailing culture helps in designing effective strategies for transformation.

76. Which of the following is a primary reason organizational cultures become resistant to change?
a. The belief that current practices are the best.
b. The organization is too large.
c. Employees are not educated enough.
d. The organization is making too much profit.

Answer: a. The belief that current practices are the best.
Explanation: Organizational inertia often stems from the belief that existing practices are optimal. This mindset can hinder the adoption of new, potentially better practices.

77. A nurse executive notices a recurring pattern of poor inter-departmental communication. Addressing this will require a change in:
a. Physical infrastructure.
b. External stakeholder management.
c. Organizational culture.
d. Hiring practices.


Answer: c. Organizational culture.
Explanation: Recurring patterns of behavior, such as poor communication, often stem from deeply rooted cultural norms. Addressing this effectively requires a change in the organizational culture.

78. A nurse executive wants to promote a culture of continuous learning. Which of the following initiatives would be least effective?
a. Encouraging attendance at workshops.
b. Offering online courses for skill development.
c. Providing financial bonuses for tenure without regard to skill enhancement.
d. Establishing a mentorship program.


Answer: c. Providing financial bonuses for tenure without regard to skill enhancement.
Explanation: Rewarding tenure without considering skill enhancement does not necessarily promote a learning culture. Instead, it might reinforce complacency.

79. What role do middle managers play in changing organizational culture?
a. They have no role as culture is determined at the top.
b. They act as a bridge between top leadership's vision and frontline implementation.
c. Their role is only to report problems, not solve them.
d. They should resist changes to maintain stability.


Answer: b. They act as a bridge between top leadership's vision and frontline implementation.
Explanation: Middle managers are crucial in translating the vision of top leadership into actionable steps and guiding frontline staff through cultural transformation.

80. Which of the following is not a typical characteristic of a toxic organizational culture?
a. Open communication.
b. Fear of retribution for mistakes.
c. Siloed departments.
d. Leadership detachment from staff concerns.

Answer: a. Open communication.
Explanation: Open communication promotes transparency and trust, while a toxic culture often suppresses open dialogue.

81. To address and change a deep-seated aspect of organizational culture, a nurse executive should:
a. Make sudden and drastic changes to shock the system.
b. Mandate changes without explaining the reasons.
c. Engage in a dialogue with staff to understand their perspectives.
d. Ignore past traditions and enforce new ones.

Answer: c. Engage in a dialogue with staff to understand their perspectives.
Explanation: Effective cultural change involves understanding and addressing the concerns and viewpoints of staff. Dialogue fosters understanding and collaboration.

82. A nurse executive seeks to change the organizational culture from hierarchical to more collaborative. Which strategy would be least effective?
a. Promoting teamwork through cross-departmental projects.
b. Implementing strict hierarchies in decision-making.
c. Offering team-building workshops.
d. Celebrating collaborative successes publicly.

Answer: b. Implementing strict hierarchies in decision-making.
Explanation: If the goal is a collaborative culture, then reinforcing strict decision-making hierarchies is counterproductive.

83. In assessing the success of cultural change initiatives, it's essential to:
a. Focus only on immediate changes.
b. Disregard employee feedback.
c. Monitor long-term trends and feedback.
d. Assume that any change is indicative of success.

Answer: c. Monitor long-term trends and feedback.
Explanation: Real cultural change is a long-term process, and its success or failure might not be immediately apparent. Continuous monitoring and feedback are essential.

84. For a cultural change initiative to succeed, the leadership should:
a. Assume that everyone will naturally adapt.
b. Communicate the need, process, and benefits of the change.
c. Avoid discussing the change to prevent panic.
d. Change only surface-level aspects and leave deep-seated norms untouched.

Answer: b. Communicate the need, process, and benefits of the change.
Explanation: Effective communication regarding why the change is happening, how it will occur, and its anticipated benefits is key to rallying staff support and understanding.

85. In a healthcare organization that operates with a flat structure, you would expect:
a. Numerous hierarchical levels and chain of commands.
b. Limited direct communication between frontline staff and leadership.
c. A decentralized decision-making process.
d. Centralized power concentrated in a few top-level executives.

Answer: c. A decentralized decision-making process.
Explanation: A flat structure often entails fewer hierarchical levels, which can lead to a more decentralized decision-making process and greater empowerment of lower-level staff.

86. A nurse executive wants to move from a functional to a matrix organizational structure. This means:
a. Eliminating all department heads.
b. Combining two distinct hierarchies: one functional and one product/project-based.
c. Consolidating all roles into a singular functional unit.
d. Separating the organization based on different medical specialties.

Answer: b. Combining two distinct hierarchies: one functional and one product/project-based.
Explanation: A matrix structure superimposes a divisional structure on a functional structure, combining both product and functional hierarchies.

87. One potential disadvantage of a divisional organizational structure in healthcare is:
a. Duplication of resources across divisions.
b. Centralization of decision-making.
c. Lack of specialization.
d. A flat hierarchy with few managerial roles.

Answer: a. Duplication of resources across divisions. Explanation: Since each division operates semi-independently in a divisional structure, there might be duplication of resources or functions across the divisions.

88. Which of the following best describes a boundaryless organizational design?
a. Strict hierarchies and limited cross-departmental collaboration.
b. An organization that works in isolation without external partnerships.
c. Fluid and flexible structures with an emphasis on eliminating barriers.
d. One that exclusively relies on virtual communication.

Answer: c. Fluid and flexible structures with an emphasis on eliminating barriers.
Explanation: A boundaryless organization seeks to remove the barriers between different parts of the organization and between the organization and its external environment.

89. In a healthcare setting, when would a team-based organizational design be most appropriate?
a. When individual work is prioritized over collaborative efforts.
b. For routine tasks that do not require interdisciplinary input.
c. When addressing complex patient care that requires multi-disciplinary teams.
d. In organizations with a rigid hierarchical culture.

Answer: c. When addressing complex patient care that requires multi-disciplinary teams.
Explanation: Team-based structures facilitate collaboration across different specialties, crucial for complex patient care scenarios requiring interdisciplinary input.

90. How can a nurse executive ensure that a hybrid organizational structure remains effective?
a. By strictly minimizing communication between different structural areas.
b. By focusing solely on one aspect of the structure and neglecting the other.
c. By clearly defining roles, responsibilities, and collaboration points.
d. By completely separating the teams under different structures.

Answer: c. By clearly defining roles, responsibilities, and collaboration points.
Explanation: For hybrid structures to be effective, clarity in roles, accountabilities, and collaboration areas is essential to prevent confusion and inefficiencies.

91. Which of the following best describes the primary focus of a functional organizational structure?
a. Product lines or projects.
b. Geographic regions.
c. Specific functions or tasks.
d. Client demographics.

Answer: c. Specific functions or tasks.
Explanation: In a functional structure, the organization is divided based on specific functions or tasks, such as nursing, pharmacy, or radiology.

92. How can a nurse executive address potential challenges in a matrix structure?
a. By eliminating one of the hierarchies to simplify.
b. By ensuring clear role delineation and effective communication channels.
c. By only relying on external consultants to make decisions.
d. By allowing teams to operate in isolation.

Answer: b. By ensuring clear role delineation and effective communication channels.
Explanation: A matrix structure's success hinges on clear role definitions and robust communication to navigate the dual hierarchies.

93. Adopting which organizational structure could potentially lead to challenges in promoting a unified organizational culture?
a. Flat structure.
b. Matrix structure.
c. Divisional structure.
d. Functional structure.

Answer: c. Divisional structure.
Explanation: Divisional structures, due to their semi-independent nature, can create silos, potentially leading to distinct cultures in each division rather than a unified organizational culture.

94. An advantage of a team-based structure in healthcare is:
a. Reduced need for communication.
b. Enhanced specialization without inter-disciplinary collaboration.
c. Increased flexibility and responsiveness to patient needs.
d. An emphasis on individual accountability over team performance.

Answer: c. Increased flexibility and responsiveness to patient needs.
Explanation: Team-based structures promote collaboration, allowing for greater flexibility and adaptability in addressing diverse patient needs.

95. A healthcare organization decides to group its resources and activities by specialization. What organizational design is this most indicative of?
a. Divisional
b. Matrix
c. Functional
d. Flat

Answer: c. Functional
Explanation: A functional design is based on grouping resources and activities by their function or specialty (e.g., nursing, radiology, administration).

96. Which design promotes the most interdepartmental collaboration due to its dual reporting relationships?
a. Functional
b. Divisional
c. Hierarchical
d. Matrix

Answer: d. Matrix
Explanation: A matrix design combines elements from both functional and divisional structures, leading to dual reporting relationships and increased collaboration.

97. A hospital is considering switching to an organizational design that emphasizes eliminating boundaries, both within the organization and with external partners. They are considering which type of structure?
a. Boundaryless
b. Hierarchical
c. Team-based
d. Functional

Answer: a. Boundaryless
Explanation: Boundaryless design is focused on removing barriers within an organization and with external entities.

98. In a networked organizational design, what is the primary focus?
a. Establishing a strict hierarchy with clear reporting lines.
b. Organizing resources around specific functions or specialties.
c. Leveraging technology to link diverse groups or teams.
d. Prioritizing individual performance over team collaboration.


Answer: c. Leveraging technology to link diverse groups or teams.
Explanation: Networked designs emphasize technology and communication tools to link various teams or departments, emphasizing flexibility and adaptability.

99. Which organizational design is best suited for an organization that offers multiple services or products and wishes to operate these services semi-independently?
a. Functional
b. Networked
c. Divisional
d. Flat


Answer: c. Divisional
Explanation: A divisional design divides the organization based on different products, services, or customer types. Each division operates semi-independently.

100. A healthcare facility that prioritizes empowering its frontline staff, reducing management layers, and promoting direct communication likely follows which organizational design?
a. Hierarchical
b. Divisional
c. Functional
d. Flat


Answer: d. Flat
Explanation: A flat structure, also known as a horizontal structure, reduces management layers and empowers frontline staff, enabling direct communication and faster decision-making.

101. In which organizational design would you likely find "communities of practice" or groups formed based on shared expertise or interests, rather than formal teams?
a. Functional
b. Adhocracy
c. Networked
d. Hierarchical

Answer: c. Networked

Explanation: In a networked design, formal and informal groups or teams, such as communities of practice, are interconnected often through technology.

102. An organization that consistently forms teams for specific projects, dissolving them upon project completion, and then forms new teams for new projects is likely utilizing which design?
a. Project-based
b. Hierarchical
c. Functional
d. Divisional

Answer: a. Project-based

Explanation: A project-based design revolves around specific projects. Teams are formed for the duration of a project and then may be dissolved.

103. Which organizational design is characterized by temporary structures, flexibility, and adaptability, often seen in start-ups or organizations undergoing innovation?
a. Hierarchical
b. Boundaryless
c. Adhocracy
d. Matrix

Answer: c. Adhocracy

Explanation: Adhocracy is characterized by adaptive, flexible structures that can change based on current needs, often seen in innovative environments.

104. For a global healthcare provider with multiple facilities worldwide, which organizational design may be most appropriate to cater to regional differences?
a. Functional
b. Geo-centric
c. Hierarchical
d. Adhocracy

Answer: b. Geo-centric

Explanation: A geo-centric or geographic design organizes the company based on regions or geographic areas, allowing for adaptation to regional differences and needs.

105. Which of the following interventions has been shown to directly improve patient care outcomes and staff job satisfaction simultaneously?
a. Increasing the number of administrators
b. Investing in cutting-edge medical equipment
c. Implementing nurse-led shared governance models
d. Introducing mandatory overtime policies

Answer: c. Implementing nurse-led shared governance models
Explanation: Nurse-led shared governance models empower frontline nurses to have a voice in decision-making processes, leading to both improved patient care and increased job satisfaction.

106. A decrease in staff turnover rates is MOST directly associated with:
a. High patient satisfaction scores
b. Administrative-driven decision making
c. Competitive compensation packages
d. Shortened shift durations

Answer: c. Competitive compensation packages
Explanation: While all factors may influence turnover rates, competitive compensation packages are a direct incentive for staff retention.

107. What is a primary way nurse executives can ensure that staffing ratios have a positive impact on patient care?
a. By hiring more junior nurses
b. By emphasizing seniority in assigning shifts
c. By matching skill level to patient acuity
d. By rotating nurses frequently between departments

Answer: c. By matching skill level to patient acuity
Explanation: Ensuring the right skill mix, where the skill level of nurses aligns with patient needs and acuity, directly affects the quality of patient care.

108. In the context of staff satisfaction, which factor is most likely to lead to nurse burnout and decreased patient care quality?
a. Regular performance evaluations
b. Access to continuing education
c. Frequent exposure to traumatic situations without support
d. Cross-training in multiple specialties

Answer: c. Frequent exposure to traumatic situations without support
Explanation: Without adequate emotional and psychological support, repeated exposure to traumatic situations can lead to nurse burnout, affecting both staff well-being and patient care.

109. Which intervention has been shown to positively impact both patient satisfaction and nurse job satisfaction?
a. Implementing a strict hierarchical structure
b. Increasing patient-to-nurse ratios
c. Encouraging multidisciplinary collaboration in patient care
d. Segregating nursing teams based on specialization

Answer: c. Encouraging multidisciplinary collaboration in patient care
Explanation: Multidisciplinary collaboration fosters a team approach, leading to holistic patient care and increased satisfaction levels for both patients and healthcare providers.

110. Nurse executive leadership that prioritizes which of the following is most likely to influence positive patient outcomes?
a. Annual reviews of nursing protocols
b. Implementation of a punitive error-reporting system
c. Regular feedback and open communication channels with frontline staff
d. Focus on cost-saving measures at the expense of resource allocation

Answer: c. Regular feedback and open communication channels with frontline staff
Explanation: Open communication fosters an environment where issues affecting patient care can be identified and addressed proactively.

111. Which factor, when prioritized, has a direct positive correlation with both patient care and staff satisfaction?
a. Strict adherence to traditional nursing roles
b. Focus on outpatient care over inpatient services
c. Emphasis on evidence-based practice
d. Reduction in staff training budgets

Answer: c. Emphasis on evidence-based practice
Explanation: Evidence-based practice ensures that patient care is based on current best evidence, leading to improved patient outcomes and increased confidence and satisfaction among staff.

112. A decrease in hospital-acquired infections can be most directly related to:
a. A decrease in patient admissions
b. Enhanced cleaning protocols
c. Increased number of administrative staff
d. Staff satisfaction with cafeteria food

Answer: b. Enhanced cleaning protocols
Explanation: Implementing and adhering to enhanced cleaning protocols is a direct measure to reduce hospital-acquired infections.

113. An effective strategy to improve staff morale and reduce feelings of powerlessness among nurses is:
a. Rotating weekly department assignments
b. Focusing solely on hard skills in training programs
c. Empowering nurses through participation in decision-making
d. Increasing the duration of shifts

Answer: c. Empowering nurses through participation in decision-making
Explanation: Empowerment through participation fosters a sense of ownership and belonging, leading to increased morale and job satisfaction.

114. What impact does frequent staff recognition and appreciation, especially in public forums, have on a healthcare organization?
a. Reduced patient wait times
b. Diminished importance of the nursing role
c. Improved staff morale and motivation
d. Increased dependence on agency staff

Answer: c. Improved staff morale and motivation
Explanation: Regular recognition and appreciation validate the contributions of staff, leading to higher morale and motivation levels.

115.St. Mercy Hospital recently underwent an organizational change by moving from a functional structure to a matrix structure. Nurse John noticed that there's been increased collaboration between departments, but there's some confusion over reporting hierarchies.

Based on the change in St. Mercy Hospital's organizational structure, which of the following challenges is Nurse John most likely observing?
a. Decreased inter-departmental communication
b. Redundancies in job roles
c. Dual reporting structures
d. A shift towards an informal communication style

Answer: c. Dual reporting structures
Explanation: In a matrix structure, employees often have dual reporting relationships – they report both to the functional manager and the product manager, which can lead to confusion.

116. Nurse Jane works in a pediatric hospital that follows a flat organizational structure. She appreciates the direct communication she has with leadership but sometimes feels overwhelmed with her broad range of responsibilities.
What is a primary advantage of the hospital's flat organizational structure?
a. Clear hierarchical reporting
b. Wider span of control
c. Reduced operational costs
d. Rapid decision-making

Answer: d. Rapid decision-making
Explanation: Flat structures often allow for quicker decision-making due to fewer hierarchical levels and more direct communication.

117. Heartbeat Clinic, a cardiac specialty clinic, is designed such that each cardiac subspecialty has its dedicated team and resources. They operate semi-independently but align with the clinic's overall mission.
Which organizational design does Heartbeat Clinic most closely resemble?
a. Matrix structure
b. Divisional structure
c. Functional structure
d. Network structure

Answer: b. Divisional structure
Explanation: In a divisional structure, each division operates semi-independently but still aligns with the organization's broader goals, similar to the cardiac subspecialties in the Heartbeat Clinic.

118. RuralCare Hospital serves a wide geographic area with limited specialized medical staff. To address various patient needs, they often collaborate with urban hospitals and specialized healthcare providers.

This approach to care most closely aligns with which organizational structure?

a. Bureaucratic
b. Matrix
c. Hierarchical
d. Network

Answer: d. Network

Explanation: Network structures involve an organization focusing on its core competencies and outsourcing other functions to other organizations or specialists.

119. Nurse Alex works at City Hospital, a large urban hospital that has departments based on functions such as nursing, pharmacy, and radiology. Each department has its specific manager.

Which organizational design is City Hospital using?

a. Divisional
b. Network
c. Functional
d. Matrix

Answer: c. Functional

Explanation: In a functional structure, the organization is divided into departments based on function or specialty, each led by a department-specific manager.

120. After a patient safety incident, River Bend Hospital decided to have a team of cross-functional members, including nurses, doctors, and pharmacists, to address the issue collectively.

This team is an example of which organizational strategy?

a. Decentralization
b. Centralization
c. Cross-functional teaming
d. Hierarchical restructuring

Answer: c. Cross-functional teaming

Explanation: Cross-functional teams consist of members from different departments or functions collaborating towards a common goal.

121. Golden Age Nursing Home has been facing challenges with delayed decisions due to a rigid hierarchical structure. The management is considering a shift to empower frontline staff with decision-making.

This shift in power dynamics is termed as:

a. Centralization
b. Decentralization
c. Functional restructuring
d. Matrixing

Answer: b. Decentralization
Explanation: Decentralization involves distributing decision-making governance closer to the patient or service user.

122. Nurse Sarah noticed that in her hospital, while the emergency department operates 24/7, certain specialty services, such as radiology, operate on fixed hours, leading to delays in patient care.

Which strategy might address this operational misalignment?

a. Implement a functional structure
b. Shift to a network structure
c. Synchronize service hours based on patient inflow
d. Introduce a divisional organizational structure

Answer: c. Synchronize service hours based on patient inflow
Explanation: Synchronizing operational hours based on patient demands or inflow can reduce waiting times and improve efficiency.

123. Metro Health Systems recently acquired a smaller hospital. The executive team is considering integrating the smaller hospital's functions into its existing structure.

Which approach might lead to challenges in cultural integration?

a. Maintaining the smaller hospital as a separate division
b. Completely absorbing and centralizing all functions
c. Forming cross-functional teams for smooth integration
d. Providing autonomy to the smaller hospital for a transition period

Answer: b. Completely absorbing and centralizing all functions
Explanation: Suddenly centralizing all functions might disregard the unique cultural aspects of the smaller hospital, leading to integration challenges.

124. Nurse Tim works in a healthcare organization where he reports to both a nursing supervisor for his clinical responsibilities and a project manager for specific projects.
Which organizational structure is this scenario indicative of?
a. Divisional
b. Functional
c. Hierarchical
d. Matrix

Answer: d. Matrix
Explanation: In a matrix structure, employees often have dual reporting relationships, in this case, to both a functional and project manager.

125. At Riverdale Hospital, Nurse Amanda observed a decline in team morale after the implementation of a new electronic health record (EHR) system. She decided to hold focus group sessions to gather feedback and address concerns.
Which leadership style is Nurse Amanda demonstrating?
a. Autocratic
b. Laissez-faire
c. Transformational
d. Transactional

Answer: c. Transformational
Explanation: Transformational leaders inspire and motivate their team by understanding their needs and addressing concerns, often leading to enhanced morale and performance.

126. Nurse James, a unit leader, strictly ensures that all protocols are followed, with a reward system for those who comply and penalties for those who don't.
Which leadership style best describes Nurse James's approach?
a. Servant leadership
b. Autocratic
c. Transformational
d. Transactional

Answer: d. Transactional
Explanation: Transactional leadership is based on a system of rewards and penalties, ensuring tasks are performed as per set protocols.

127. At Sunshine Clinic, Nurse Laura noticed a team member struggling with a personal issue. She took the initiative to adjust his schedule and connected him with counseling services.

This action is most indicative of which leadership quality?
a. Task-oriented behavior
b. Charisma
c. Emotional intelligence
d. Professional authority

Answer: c. Emotional intelligence
Explanation: Recognizing and addressing team members' emotional needs showcases a leader's emotional intelligence.

128. Nurse Mike always emphasizes the "why" behind any change or protocol, ensuring his team understands the purpose and is motivated to adopt the change.
Which leadership style is Nurse Mike likely using?
a. Bureaucratic
b. Transformational
c. Situational
d. Laissez-faire

Answer: b. Transformational. Explanation: Transformational leaders focus on the bigger picture, inspiring and motivating their team by ensuring they understand the "why" behind actions.

129. In the pediatric wing, Nurse Anna often consults her team before making decisions, valuing the collective input of all members.
This is characteristic of which leadership style?
a. Autocratic
b. Democratic
c. Transactional
d. Charismatic

Answer: b. Democratic  Explanation: Democratic leaders often seek input from their team members before finalizing decisions.

130. Nurse Benjamin leads a diverse team. He understands the cultural and personal differences among team members and leverages their unique strengths for patient care.
Which leadership quality is Nurse Benjamin strongly demonstrating?
a. Technical prowess
b. Cultural intelligence
c. Command authority
d. Task orientation

Answer: b. Cultural intelligence
Explanation: Recognizing and appreciating cultural differences and leveraging them for improved outcomes shows a high level of cultural intelligence.

131. Nurse Clara was appointed as the unit leader for the emergency department during an unexpected crisis. Her ability to adapt her leadership style based on the situation was praised. Which leadership style does this depict?
a. Situational
b. Transformational
c. Autocratic
d. Bureaucratic

Answer: a. Situational
Explanation: Situational leaders adapt their style based on the demands of a particular situation.

132. Nurse Derek has a hands-off approach, trusting his team to make decisions and intervene only when necessary.
What leadership style is he exhibiting?
a. Laissez-faire
b. Autocratic
c. Democratic
d. Transformational

Answer: a. Laissez-faire
Explanation: Laissez-faire leaders have a more hands-off approach, allowing team members to make decisions and intervening minimally.

133. Nurse Elaine always prioritizes the needs of her team, ensuring they have the necessary resources and training. She believes that by serving them, the quality of patient care will improve.
This approach aligns with which leadership style?
a. Servant leadership
b. Autocratic
c. Transactional
d. Charismatic

Answer: a. Servant leadership
Explanation: Servant leaders prioritize the needs of their team, believing that by doing so, the broader objectives of the organization will be achieved.

134. Nurse Frank, despite being the head of the department, often spends time with new nurses, mentoring them, and understanding their challenges.
This is indicative of which leadership quality?
a. Technical expertise
b. Autonomy
c. Emotional intelligence
d. Approachability

Answer: d. Approachability
Explanation: Leaders who are accessible and willing to spend time mentoring and understanding their team's challenges are considered approachable.

135. Which leadership theory emphasizes the importance of leaders adapting their style based on the situation and the maturity level of their subordinates?
a. Path-Goal Theory
b. Transformational Leadership Theory
c. Situational Leadership Theory
d. Trait Theory

Answer: c. Situational Leadership Theory
Explanation: The Situational Leadership Theory posits that leaders should adjust their style based on the situation and the readiness or maturity of their team members.

136. Leaders who prioritize the needs and well-being of their team members, believing that by serving them, the broader objectives of the organization will be achieved, are adhering to which leadership style?
a. Autocratic Leadership
b. Servant Leadership
c. Laissez-faire Leadership
d. Transactional Leadership

Answer: b. Servant Leadership
Explanation: Servant Leadership is a style where the leader prioritizes the needs and growth of their team members above all else, believing this approach will ultimately benefit the entire organization.

137. Which leadership style is characterized by a leader who gives clear directions and expects strict compliance from team members?
a. Democratic Leadership
b. Transformational Leadership
c. Autocratic Leadership
d. Situational Leadership

Answer: c. Autocratic Leadership
Explanation: Autocratic leaders make decisions unilaterally and expect team members to comply without input.

138. In which leadership theory do leaders motivate followers by appealing to their higher ideals and moral values?
a. Contingency Theory
b. Transformational Leadership Theory
c. Trait Theory
d. Path-Goal Theory

Answer: b. Transformational Leadership Theory
Explanation: Transformational leaders inspire and motivate followers by appealing to their higher ideals, values, and emotions.

139. Which leadership style involves a leader who often steps back, allowing team members to take charge and make decisions, intervening minimally?
a. Servant Leadership
b. Laissez-faire Leadership
c. Transactional Leadership
d. Autocratic Leadership

Answer: b. Laissez-faire Leadership
Explanation: Laissez-faire leaders tend to have a more hands-off approach, allowing team members more freedom in decision-making.

140. Leaders who focus on transactions, using a system of rewards and punishments to motivate team members, are adhering to which style of leadership?
a. Transformational Leadership
b. Servant Leadership
c. Transactional Leadership
d. Democratic Leadership

Answer: c. Transactional Leadership
Explanation: Transactional Leadership is based on a system of rewards and punishments to motivate team members and ensure tasks are performed.

141. Which leadership theory suggests that successful leadership is based on a match between a leader's style and the specific demands of a situation?
a. Trait Theory
b. Contingency Theory
c. Path-Goal Theory
d. Transformational Leadership Theory

Answer: b. Contingency Theory
Explanation: Contingency Theory posits that optimal leadership effectiveness results from a match between the leader's style and the demands of the situation.

142. Which leadership theory posits that leaders provide followers with resources and support to achieve goals, altering their style based on the task and the individual's capabilities?
a. Trait Theory
b. Transformational Leadership Theory
c. Path-Goal Theory
d. Situational Leadership Theory

Answer: c. Path-Goal Theory
Explanation: Path-Goal Theory focuses on how leaders can help followers achieve their goals by providing direction, support, and resources, adjusting based on the task and individual.

143. Which leadership theory emphasizes that specific characteristics and traits are inherent in great leaders?
a. Trait Theory
b. Path-Goal Theory
c. Contingency Theory
d. Transformational Leadership Theory

Answer: a. Trait Theory
Explanation: Trait Theory suggests that certain individual characteristics and traits are inherent in leaders or contribute significantly to leadership effectiveness.

144. Which leadership style involves a leader who values collective input, making decisions that are in the best interest of the majority?
a. Democratic Leadership
b. Autocratic Leadership
c. Transactional Leadership
d. Laissez-faire Leadership

Answer: a. Democratic Leadership
Explanation: Democratic leaders value the input of their team members and often make decisions based on the consensus or what's in the best interest of the majority.

145. A nurse leader encourages her staff to explore innovative solutions and places significant emphasis on personal and professional growth. Which type of leadership style is she most likely utilizing?
a. Transactional Leadership
b. Autocratic Leadership
c. Transformational Leadership
d. Laissez-faire Leadership

Answer: c. Transformational Leadership. Explanation: Transformational leaders inspire and motivate their team, promoting innovation, and placing a high emphasis on personal and professional growth.

146. Within the context of healthcare leadership, which theory emphasizes the importance of social interactions, empowerment, and increasing the collective capability of the staff?
a. Shared Leadership
b. Trait Theory
c. Path-Goal Theory
d. Contingency Theory

Answer: a. Shared Leadership. Explanation: Shared Leadership focuses on social interactions and collective empowerment, emphasizing team collaboration and joint responsibility.

147. In a busy clinical setting, a nurse manager rewards staff with bonuses for high patient satisfaction scores and gives warnings to those with low scores. This approach is an example of which leadership style?
a. Democratic Leadership
b. Transformational Leadership
c. Laissez-faire Leadership
d. Transactional Leadership

Answer: d. Transactional Leadership
Explanation: Transactional leaders operate on an exchange basis, providing rewards for good performance and penalties for poor performance.

148. A nurse leader believes that specific inherent traits and characteristics lead to effective leadership. This belief aligns with which leadership theory?
a. Trait Theory
b. Path-Goal Theory
c. Shared Leadership
d. Transformational Leadership

Answer: a. Trait Theory
Explanation: Trait Theory posits that specific individual characteristics and inherent traits determine leadership effectiveness.

149. Within the context of healthcare, which leadership theory suggests that effective leadership is not solely a product of the situation or the leader's traits but a combination of both?
a. Shared Leadership
b. Contingency Theory
c. Transactional Leadership
d. Path-Goal Theory

Answer: b. Contingency Theory
Explanation: Contingency Theory posits that leadership effectiveness results from the congruence between a leader's style and the demands of the situation.

150. A healthcare executive emphasizes the importance of shared decision-making and flattening the hierarchical structure. This approach is closely associated with:
a. Laissez-faire Leadership
b. Democratic Leadership
c. Shared Leadership
d. Autocratic Leadership

Answer: c. Shared Leadership
Explanation: Shared Leadership promotes collective decision-making and often emphasizes reducing hierarchical structures to promote team collaboration.

151. A clinical nurse specialist motivates the team by conveying a strong vision, fostering trust, and challenging them to think critically. This style resonates with which leadership approach?
a. Transactional Leadership
b. Autocratic Leadership
c. Transformational Leadership
d. Democratic Leadership

Answer: c. Transformational Leadership
Explanation: Transformational leaders motivate and inspire by conveying a strong vision, building trust, and challenging their teams to innovate and think critically.

152. Which leadership theory in healthcare focuses on maximizing the strengths of each team member and believes that leadership roles can shift based on the situation?
a. Contingency Theory
b. Shared Leadership
c. Transformational Leadership
d. Trait Theory

Answer: b. Shared Leadership
Explanation: Shared Leadership emphasizes the importance of each team member's strengths and believes that leadership roles can be dynamic based on specific situations.

153. In a hospital setting, a nurse manager sets clear guidelines, expects strict adherence, and rewards or penalizes based on performance metrics. This approach mirrors:
a. Transactional Leadership
b. Transformational Leadership
c. Democratic Leadership
d. Laissez-faire Leadership

Answer: a. Transactional Leadership

Explanation: Transactional leadership is characterized by clear guidelines and an emphasis on rewards and penalties based on performance metrics.

154. A nurse leader frequently involves the team in decision-making processes and promotes a culture where everyone's opinions are valued. This approach is indicative of:
a. Laissez-faire Leadership
b. Democratic Leadership
c. Autocratic Leadership
d. Transactional Leadership

Answer: b. Democratic Leadership

Explanation: Democratic leaders involve their teams in decision-making processes and foster an environment where everyone's opinions are valued.

155. A nurse leader recognizes a persistent issue with missed medication doses during the night shift. What critical leadership skill should they prioritize to address this issue?
a. Decision-making
b. Technical competence in medication administration
c. Conflict resolution
d. Strategic visioning

Answer: a. Decision-making

Explanation: While all the options are valuable leadership skills, decision-making is crucial to identify solutions and implement interventions for the recognized issue.

156. During a team meeting, a staff nurse openly criticizes a new policy. The nurse executive responds by listening and then seeking clarity on the concerns. Which leadership skill is the executive displaying?
a. Emotional intelligence
b. Technical skill
c. Autonomy
d. Time management

Answer: a. Emotional intelligence

Explanation: Emotional intelligence is vital in understanding and managing both one's emotions and those of the team. Actively listening and seeking clarity demonstrates high emotional intelligence.

157. When preparing for potential future challenges in healthcare delivery, which leadership skill is essential for a nurse executive?
a. Tactical proficiency
b. Clinical expertise
c. Futuristic thinking
d. Micro-management

Answer: c. Futuristic thinking
Explanation: Futuristic thinking allows leaders to anticipate and prepare for potential future challenges, ensuring that the organization is ready for changes in healthcare delivery.

158. In a rapidly changing healthcare environment, which leadership skill is crucial for a nurse leader to ensure the team remains updated and competent?
a. Strong clinical background
b. Adaptability
c. Autocratic decision-making
d. Budgeting

Answer: b. Adaptability
Explanation: The healthcare environment is dynamic. Leaders must be adaptable to manage change effectively and ensure their teams remain competent and updated.

159. A nurse leader is tasked with developing a program to improve patient satisfaction scores. Which skill would be crucial in ensuring that the team buys into this new initiative?
a. Influencing
b. Technical knowledge of patient care
c. Task delegation
d. Autonomy

Answer: a. Influencing
Explanation: To get team buy-in for new initiatives, leaders must influence their team, ensuring understanding and commitment to the program.

160. During a budget deficit, a nurse executive needs to make decisions about resource allocation without compromising patient care. Which leadership skill is being tested the most?
a. Clinical knowledge
b. Conflict resolution
c. Financial acumen
d. Time management

Answer: c. Financial acumen
Explanation: Financial acumen is essential when making decisions related to budgeting and resource allocation, especially during financial constraints.

161. Which essential leadership skill ensures that a nurse leader effectively communicates the organization's vision, ensuring alignment with the team's daily activities?
a. Futuristic thinking
b. Communication
c. Task delegation
d. Clinical expertise

Answer: b. Communication
Explanation: Effective communication is crucial for transmitting the organization's vision and ensuring that the team's activities align with that vision.

162. A nurse executive mentors a budding nurse leader, guiding them through challenges and sharing valuable insights. This is an example of which leadership skill?
a. Coaching and mentoring
b. Conflict resolution
c. Clinical expertise
d. Task delegation

Answer: a. Coaching and mentoring
Explanation: Coaching and mentoring are vital leadership skills that involve guiding less experienced individuals, helping them navigate challenges, and sharing insights.

163. During a challenging period for the healthcare facility, the nurse leader consistently showcases optimism and motivation, instilling hope in the team. Which leadership skill is this?
a. Resilience
b. Clinical skills
c. Time management
d. Task delegation

Answer: a. Resilience
Explanation: Resilience enables leaders to bounce back from challenges, maintain optimism, and instill hope in their teams during tough times.

164. A nurse leader frequently assesses the team's strengths and weaknesses, aligns tasks based on expertise, and ensures efficient workflow. Which leadership skill is this indicative of?
a. Time management
b. Resource allocation
c. Clinical knowledge
d. Decision-making

Answer: b. Resource allocation
Explanation: Efficiently assessing team strengths and aligning tasks to optimize workflow is an example of effective resource allocation.

165. Two senior nurses have a disagreement about the implementation of a new protocol. The nurse executive steps in and decides to implement the protocol as per one of the nurse's suggestions, without seeking the other nurse's input. This approach to conflict resolution can be described as:
a. Collaborative
b. Avoidant
c. Accommodating
d. Competitive

Answer: d. Competitive
Explanation: The competitive approach involves pursuing one's viewpoint at another's expense. It's authoritative in nature and may resolve conflicts quickly, but it can also cause resentment.

166. A nurse executive holds a meeting to discuss a recent disagreement between two departments. She ensures that both parties voice their concerns and together they reach a mutual agreement. This style of conflict resolution is known as:
a. Compromising
b. Collaborative
c. Obliging
d. Avoidant

Answer: b. Collaborative
Explanation: The collaborative approach aims to meet the needs of all parties involved. It seeks a win-win solution by addressing the concerns and requirements of each side.

167. During a heated team meeting, a nurse leader recognizes the escalating tension and decides to table the discussion for another day. This is an example of which conflict resolution technique?
a. Smoothing
b. Avoidance
c. Compromising
d. Confrontation

Answer: b. Avoidance
Explanation: Avoidance involves postponing or sidestepping conflict. It might provide a temporary solution but can lead to unresolved issues in the long run.

168. A nurse leader consistently ensures that any interpersonal conflicts among team members are discussed in private settings to maintain team morale. This strategy emphasizes the importance of:
a. Open communication
b. Maintaining team dignity
c. Collaborative decision-making
d. Hierarchical decision-making

Answer: b. Maintaining team dignity
Explanation: Addressing conflicts in private settings ensures that individuals feel respected and maintains the dignity of the team as a whole.

169. In a conflict about resource allocation, a nurse executive decides to split the available resources equally between two departments, even though neither solution fully addresses the departments' needs. This conflict resolution style is:
a. Avoidant
b. Competitive
c. Compromising
d. Collaborative

Answer: c. Compromising
Explanation: The compromising style aims for a quick resolution by finding a middle ground. While it may not fully satisfy all parties, it can be an effective temporary solution.

170. To preemptively address potential conflicts, a nurse executive sets clear expectations and roles for all team members. This strategy focuses on:
a. Conflict suppression
b. Proactive conflict management
c. Reactive conflict resolution
d. Passive conflict avoidance

Answer: b. Proactive conflict management
Explanation: By setting clear expectations and roles ahead of time, the executive is proactively managing potential areas of conflict.

171. A nurse leader notices a recurring conflict between two staff members. Instead of directly intervening, she brings in a neutral third-party mediator to help. This approach is known as:
a. Arbitration
b. Collaboration
c. Mediation
d. Avoidance

Answer: c. Mediation
Explanation: Mediation involves a neutral third party helping conflicting parties to come to an agreement. It's different from arbitration where the third party makes a decision.

172. After a disagreement in a team meeting, a nurse leader acknowledges the diverse viewpoints and suggests they all take a short break before reconvening. This technique is:
a. Smoothing
b. Collaborative
c. Avoidant
d. Compromising

Answer: a. Smoothing
Explanation: Smoothing involves acknowledging differences and temporarily alleviating tension, with the intention of addressing the conflict at a later time.

173. In a team conflict, a nurse leader gathers data from all involved parties and makes an informed decision that she believes will best benefit patient care. This approach is grounded in:
a. Evidence-based decision-making
b. Hierarchical resolution
c. Compromising
d. Collaboration

Answer: a. Evidence-based decision-making
Explanation: By gathering data and basing the decision on evidence, the leader is employing evidence-based decision-making to resolve the conflict.

174. A nurse executive brings together two conflicting parties to openly discuss and understand each other's perspectives, without pushing for an immediate solution. This method is known as:
a. Dialogue
b. Confrontation
c. Mediation
d. Compromising

Answer: a. Dialogue
Explanation: Dialogue encourages open communication, understanding, and empathy, allowing parties to gain insight into each other's viewpoints without the immediate pressure to resolve the issue.

175. A nurse executive aims to involve the nursing staff in the decision-making process regarding new workflow policies. This approach is a reflection of:
a. Autocratic decision-making
b. Participative decision-making
c. Delegative decision-making
d. Reactive decision-making

Answer: b. Participative decision-making
Explanation: Participative decision-making involves including team members in the decision-making process. It can boost morale and acceptance of decisions.

176. In a situation where immediate decisions are needed in a crisis, the most appropriate decision-making style is:
a. Collaborative
b. Autocratic
c. Laissez-faire
d. Democratic

Answer: b. Autocratic
Explanation: In crises, there might not be time for broad consultation. An autocratic approach allows for rapid decisions by a single authority figure.

177. A nurse manager assigns a charge nurse to create a new shift schedule but retains the right to make the final approval. This process is an example of:
a. Empowerment
b. Abdication
c. Delegation
d. Negotiation

Answer: c. Delegation
Explanation: Delegation involves assigning responsibility to another while retaining ultimate accountability.

178. A nurse leader facilitates a meeting where team members discuss the pros and cons of a decision and come to a consensus. This approach showcases the use of:
a. Negotiation
b. Delegation
c. Autocratic decision-making
d. Empowerment

Answer: a. Negotiation
Explanation: Negotiation is a dialogue between parties aimed at reaching a consensus or agreement.

179. The act of providing team members with tools, training, resources, authority, and opportunity to manage their own work is referred to as:
a. Delegation
b. Negotiation
c. Empowerment
d. Autocratic decision-making

Answer: c. Empowerment
Explanation: Empowerment involves giving individuals the means and authority to make decisions and take actions autonomously.

180. A nurse executive who typically asks for input from her team but makes the final decision by herself is employing which decision-making style?
a. Autocratic
b. Democratic
c. Laissez-faire
d. Consultative

Answer: d. Consultative
Explanation: A consultative decision-making style involves seeking input from others but the leader makes the final decision.

181. A nurse leader who avoids making decisions and allows the team to decide on their own is using which decision-making style?
a. Autocratic
b. Democratic
c. Laissez-faire
d. Consultative

Answer: c. Laissez-faire
Explanation: Laissez-faire leadership allows team members to make decisions without much guidance or intervention.

182. Two departments are in disagreement about resource allocation. The nurse executive brings representatives from both departments to the table to find a middle ground. This approach is an example of:
a. Delegation
b. Empowerment
c. Abdication
d. Negotiation

Answer: d. Negotiation
Explanation: Negotiation involves dialogue between parties to find a common ground or agreement.

183. A nurse leader assigns a task to a junior nurse and also provides the authority to make certain decisions regarding that task. However, the leader is still ultimately responsible for the outcome. This process is known as:
a. Empowerment
b. Abdication
c. Negotiation
d. Delegation

Answer: d. Delegation
Explanation: Delegation involves giving someone else the authority to perform a task, but the person who delegated remains accountable.

184. In preparation for implementing a new hospital policy, a nurse executive schedules sessions where nurses can provide feedback and express concerns. By doing so, the executive is:
a. Abdicating responsibility
b. Delegating the task
c. Empowering the nursing staff
d. Using autocratic decision-making

Answer: c. Empowering the nursing staff
Explanation: By actively seeking feedback and involving nurses in the policy discussions, the executive is empowering them and acknowledging their vital role in the process.

185. A nurse executive is preparing to implement an electronic health record (EHR) system in a facility that has always used paper documentation. The first step in ensuring a successful transition is to:
a. Choose the most advanced EHR system available.
b. Train the staff on the new EHR system.
c. Understand the unique needs and challenges of the facility.
d. Consult with EHR vendors for the best deals.

Answer: c. Understand the unique needs and challenges of the facility.
Explanation: Before any change, understanding the context in which the change will occur is crucial. The unique challenges and needs of the facility will inform the best choices moving forward.

186. The primary objective of using Lewin's Change Management Model in a healthcare setting is to:
a. Secure top-down management support.
b. Develop a robust training program.
c. Understand the change process as unfreeze, change, and refreeze.
d. Increase budget allocation for the change initiative.

Answer: c. Understand the change process as unfreeze, change, and refreeze.
Explanation: Lewin's model breaks change into three stages: unfreezing (preparing for the change), changing (making the change), and refreezing (solidifying the change).

187. During the rollout of a new clinical procedure, the nursing staff expresses concerns and resistance. A transformational nurse leader should:
a. Tell the staff that the change is mandatory and non-negotiable.
b. Listen to the staff's concerns and involve them in finding solutions.
c. Implement the procedure as planned without delay.
d. Inform the staff that the decision has been made at the top level and must be followed.

Answer: b. Listen to the staff's concerns and involve them in finding solutions.
Explanation: Transformational leaders encourage open communication and collaboration. Listening to concerns can provide insights and foster buy-in.

188. When using Kotter's 8-Step Change Model in healthcare, which of the following is the first step?
a. Forming a strategic vision.
b. Enlisting a volunteer army.
c. Communicating the vision.
d. Creating a sense of urgency.

Answer: d. Creating a sense of urgency.
Explanation: Kotter's model begins with creating a sense of urgency, ensuring stakeholders recognize the need for change.

189. A common reason for resistance to change in healthcare settings is:
a. Excessive communication from leadership.
b. Too many resources available for staff.
c. Fear of the unknown and concern about competency post-change.
d. Quick implementation without delays.

Answer: c. Fear of the unknown and concern about competency post-change.
Explanation: Staff often resist change due to uncertainty and fear about their roles and abilities after the change.

190. After implementing a new patient care model, a nurse executive realizes that there's significant pushback from the nursing staff. An appropriate next step is to:
a. Terminate non-compliant staff.
b. Continue with the plan without addressing concerns.
c. Re-evaluate the model, gather feedback, and adjust as necessary.
d. Introduce another new model immediately.

Answer: c. Re-evaluate the model, gather feedback, and adjust as necessary.
Explanation: Feedback is crucial in change management. If there's pushback, re-evaluation and adjustment based on feedback can help ensure success.

191. For successful change management, which of the following is essential?
a. Keeping the decision-making process only at the executive level.
b. Implementing changes as quickly as possible.
c. Ensuring clear and consistent communication throughout the process.
d. Avoiding feedback loops to prevent confusion.

Answer: c. Ensuring clear and consistent communication throughout the process.
Explanation: Effective communication helps everyone understand the why, what, and how of the change, and is crucial for buy-in and successful implementation.

192. During a significant organizational change, which of the following stakeholder groups should be involved to ensure a holistic approach?
a. Only the nursing staff.
b. Only the top management.
c. Nursing staff, physicians, support staff, and patients.
d. Only the nurse executive team.

Answer: c. Nursing staff, physicians, support staff, and patients.
Explanation: Involving a wide range of stakeholders ensures diverse perspectives are considered, leading to more holistic and effective change.

193. A nurse executive notes that while the hospital's recent change initiative is conceptually sound, there's a lack of engagement and enthusiasm among the staff. A potential remedy for this is:
a. Reducing the number of staff meetings to save time.
b. Offering financial incentives for rapid adoption of the change.
c. Involving staff in the change process and recognizing their contributions.
d. Informing staff that non-adherence will lead to disciplinary action.

Answer: c. Involving staff in the change process and recognizing their contributions.
Explanation: Engagement often improves when staff feel they're a valuable part of the change process and when their efforts are acknowledged.

194. A healthcare facility is transitioning to a new IT system. To ensure smooth adaptation, the nurse executive should prioritize:
a. Immediate discontinuation of the old system.
b. Comprehensive training and support for all users.
c. Limited access to the system for the first month.
d. Introduction of the new system in the executive departments first.

Answer: b. Comprehensive training and support for all users.
Explanation: Proper training and support ensure users are comfortable with the new system, reducing errors and resistance.

195. A nurse executive decides to implement a new nursing care model. To secure staff buy-in, which strategy is the most effective at the outset?
a. Establish mandatory training sessions.
b. Seek feedback only after full implementation.
c. Explain the consequences of not adopting the new model.
d. Involve frontline staff in planning and decision-making processes.

Answer: d. Involve frontline staff in planning and decision-making processes.
Explanation: Actively involving staff from the start fosters ownership and reduces resistance, as they feel their perspectives are valued.

196. In the middle of a major change initiative, some team members are highly resistant. What should a nurse executive primarily consider when addressing this resistance?
a. The individual personalities of the resistors.
b. The underlying concerns and reasons for the resistance.
c. The influence of resistant members on others.
d. The feasibility of replacing resistant members.

Answer: b. The underlying concerns and reasons for the resistance.
Explanation: Addressing the root causes of resistance helps to tailor interventions effectively. By understanding concerns, leaders can offer solutions or clarify misunderstandings.

197. After a significant change has been implemented, a key strategy to ensure its success and sustainability is:
a. Taking disciplinary actions against non-compliers.
b. Discontinuing old methods and practices immediately.
c. Providing ongoing training and support.
d. Introducing another significant change to maintain momentum.

Answer: c. Providing ongoing training and support.
Explanation: Continuous training ensures that staff remain competent and comfortable with the change, reducing the likelihood of reverting to old methods.

198. To evaluate the effectiveness of a newly implemented change, what is the most important aspect a nurse executive should consider?
a. The ease of implementation.
b. The opinions of the management team.
c. Tangible outcomes related to patient care and staff satisfaction.
d. The speed at which the change was adopted.

Answer: c. Tangible outcomes related to patient care and staff satisfaction.
Explanation: While various factors are essential, the impact on patient care and staff satisfaction provides a direct measure of a change's effectiveness.

199. A nurse executive is aware that not every team member will support a proposed change. A proactive approach to mitigate potential resistance is to:
a. Inform the team that resistance will not be tolerated.
b. Only involve team members who are known to be supportive.
c. Address potential concerns transparently before they become bigger issues.
d. Keep details about the change limited to prevent misinformation.

Answer: c. Address potential concerns transparently before they become bigger issues.
Explanation: Addressing concerns proactively helps to alleviate fears and can prevent misinformation and rumors from taking root.

200. During the evaluation phase of a change initiative, a nurse executive notes that while the change has brought about improved patient outcomes, the nursing staff seems highly stressed. The next step should be:
a. Ignore staff stress as patient outcomes are more critical.
b. Revert to the old methods to ensure staff satisfaction.
c. Investigate the causes of the stress and consider adjustments to the change.
d. Introduce relaxation techniques for the staff.

Answer: c. Investigate the causes of the stress and consider adjustments to the change.
Explanation: While improved patient outcomes are vital, staff well-being is equally essential. The goal should be to find a balance where both patients and staff benefit.

201. One of the frontline managers is very vocal about their disagreement with a proposed change. What's the best way for a nurse executive to handle this situation?
a. Request the manager's resignation for undermining the initiative.
b. Ignore the manager's concerns and proceed.
c. Engage the manager in a constructive dialogue to understand their concerns.
d. Limit the manager's involvement in future change initiatives.

Answer: c. Engage the manager in a constructive dialogue to understand their concerns.
Explanation: Open communication can lead to a mutual understanding, and the manager's insights might offer valuable feedback for the initiative.

202. A newly implemented change isn't producing the desired results. A nurse executive should:
a. Wait for a more extended period to see if outcomes improve.
b. Discontinue the change and revert to the old system.
c. Re-evaluate, adjust the strategy, and monitor closely.
d. Seek external consultants to manage the process.

Answer: c. Re-evaluate, adjust the strategy, and monitor closely.
Explanation: Continuous evaluation and adjustment are vital in change management. If a change isn't producing desired outcomes, leaders should adjust as necessary.

203. To create a culture where change is embraced rather than feared, a nurse executive should prioritize:
a. Strict hierarchies and clear chains of command.
b. A punitive approach to mistakes.
c. Open communication and a learning environment.
d. A top-down approach to decision-making.

Answer: c. Open communication and a learning environment.
Explanation: An open and learning-oriented culture makes it easier for team members to adapt to and accept changes.

204. After implementing a change, what metric is not typically used to evaluate its effectiveness?
a. Financial savings.
b. Increase in management's power.
c. Patient satisfaction scores.
d. Staff feedback.

Answer: b. Increase in management's power.
Explanation: While various metrics can be used to evaluate a change, an increase in management's power isn't typically a metric tied to effective change in healthcare settings.

205. A nurse executive is implementing succession planning for nursing leadership roles. An important first step is to:
a. Select potential candidates based on years of service.
b. Identify critical roles and their core competencies.
c. Announce the succession planning to all staff members.
d. Start conducting training sessions on advanced leadership.

Answer: b. Identify critical roles and their core competencies.
Explanation: Recognizing essential roles and defining their required competencies helps target development efforts and select suitable candidates for those roles.

206. In the context of succession planning, which of these actions is most effective in developing potential leaders from within the nursing staff?
a. Regularly rotating staff through various roles.
b. Promoting the most senior nurse to leadership roles.
c. Offering financial incentives for those who take on extra responsibilities.
d. Providing only classroom-based leadership training.

Answer: a. Regularly rotating staff through various roles.
Explanation: Rotational assignments expose staff to various aspects of operations and roles, which builds a broad base of experience and uncovers leadership potential.

207. A successful succession plan for nurse leadership should be:
a. Static and based on current needs.
b. Confidential and known only to top management.
c. Fluid, revisited regularly, and adaptable.
d. Solely based on performance evaluations.

Answer: c. Fluid, revisited regularly, and adaptable.
Explanation: Organizational needs and staff competencies evolve. A good succession plan should be regularly updated to remain relevant and effective.

208. When considering succession planning, a nurse executive identifies a high-potential nurse for a leadership role. What's the next appropriate step?
a. Fast-track the nurse for a promotion.
b. Inform the nurse's colleagues about the potential promotion.
c. Create a tailored development plan for the nurse.
d. Send the nurse for an external leadership course immediately.

Answer: c. Create a tailored development plan for the nurse.
Explanation: A personalized development plan ensures that the potential leader acquires the necessary skills and experiences to succeed in future leadership roles.

209. Why is mentoring an essential component of succession planning?
a. It allows senior leaders to delegate their tasks.
b. It ensures that only the most experienced staff are promoted.
c. It fosters knowledge transfer and professional growth.
d. It reduces the workload of senior leaders.

Answer: c. It fosters knowledge transfer and professional growth.
Explanation: Mentoring ensures that valuable insights, experiences, and institutional knowledge are passed down, helping potential leaders to grow in their roles.

210. What is a potential risk of not having a succession plan in place?
a. Increased reliance on external hires when leadership vacancies arise.
b. An oversupply of competent internal candidates for leadership roles.
c. Reduced training and development costs.
d. Increased job satisfaction among senior leaders.

Answer: a. Increased reliance on external hires when leadership vacancies arise.
Explanation: Without a succession plan, there might be a lack of ready internal candidates, leading to a dependence on external hires, which may not always align with the organization's culture.

211. For succession planning to be effective, it requires:
a. The involvement of human resources only.
b. A focus only on senior leadership roles.
c. Commitment from the entire organization, including top management.
d. Immediate promotions for high-performing staff.

Answer: c. Commitment from the entire organization, including top management.
Explanation: Succession planning's success hinges on organization-wide commitment, ensuring alignment, resources, and support for potential leaders.

212. During the implementation of a succession plan, it's observed that many potential leaders are leaving the organization. What should be the nurse executive's priority?
a. Reevaluate the plan and seek feedback from potential leaders.
b. Increase the salaries of potential leaders.
c. Accelerate promotions to retain potential leaders.
d. Focus on hiring external candidates with leadership potential.

Answer: a. Reevaluate the plan and seek feedback from potential leaders.
Explanation: Understanding the reasons behind departures is crucial. Feedback can provide insights and guide adjustments to better support and retain potential leaders.

213. When aligning succession planning with organizational strategy, a nurse executive should:
a. Focus on the present needs of the organization.
b. Prioritize external training programs.
c. Align potential leaders' development with the organization's future direction.
d. Only consider the preferences of the board of directors.

Answer: c. Align potential leaders' development with the organization's future direction.
Explanation: Succession planning should be forward-looking, ensuring that future leaders have the skills and competencies to lead in the organization's intended direction.

214. A nurse executive is assessing the effectiveness of the current succession plan. Which metric would be least relevant?
a. Retention rates of identified potential leaders.
b. Feedback from mentors and mentees.
c. Number of external leadership hires.
d. Current patient satisfaction scores.

Answer: d. Current patient satisfaction scores.
Explanation: While patient satisfaction is crucial, it doesn't directly reflect the effectiveness of a succession plan. The other options offer more direct insights into the plan's success.

215. In the context of nursing leadership, why is the use of case studies considered crucial?
a. They provide a theoretical foundation for nursing practices.
b. They offer opportunities for memorization and rote learning.
c. They deliver real-world examples that foster critical thinking.
d. They primarily focus on the historical aspects of nursing.

Answer: c. They deliver real-world examples that foster critical thinking.
Explanation: Case studies present real-life scenarios, allowing nursing leaders to analyze situations, make decisions, and reflect on outcomes, promoting critical thinking skills.

216. A nurse executive is implementing a new electronic health record (EHR) system. To ensure smooth integration, she refers to a case study from a similar institution. This is an example of:
a. Benchmarking.
b. Ethnography.
c. Cross-sectional analysis.
d. A Delphi study.

Answer: a. Benchmarking.
Explanation: Benchmarking involves comparing one's own organization to others (often through case studies) to identify best practices and improve performance.

217. When developing a case study for educational purposes, which component is essential?
a. Hypothetical scenarios.
b. A focus on past practices.
c. Detailed background information and context.
d. Broad generalizations.

Answer: c. Detailed background information and context.
Explanation: For a case study to be effective, it should provide ample background and context, allowing individuals to understand and analyze the situation comprehensively.

218. Which of the following best illustrates the primary strength of case studies in nursing leadership training?
a. Providing a comprehensive review of all possible scenarios.
b. Allowing for exploration of complex, real-world problems in depth.
c. Offering a controlled environment to test hypotheses.
d. Delivering concise summaries of vast topics.

Answer: b. Allowing for exploration of complex, real-world problems in depth.
Explanation: Case studies delve deep into specific issues or scenarios, providing richness and depth, which fosters a comprehensive understanding.

219. When critiquing a case study, what aspect should a nurse executive pay close attention to?
a. The length of the study.
b. The number of references used.
c. The representativeness and generalizability of the findings.
d. The use of colorful charts and diagrams.

Answer: c. The representativeness and generalizability of the findings.
Explanation: While case studies provide in-depth insights, it's essential to consider if the findings are representative and can be generalized to other settings.

220. A nurse executive reads a case study about a successful intervention implemented in a rural clinic. Before applying the intervention in her urban hospital, she should:
a. Assume that what worked in one setting will work in another.
b. Replicate the intervention without any adjustments.
c. Analyze the contextual differences and adapt the intervention accordingly.
d. Focus solely on the end results presented in the case study.

Answer: c. Analyze the contextual differences and adapt the intervention accordingly.
Explanation: Context matters. Differences between rural and urban settings can significantly influence the applicability of an intervention.

221. Which of the following methods would be the least effective when gathering data for a nursing leadership case study?
a. In-depth interviews.
b. Direct observation.
c. Random number generation.
d. Document analysis.

Answer: c. Random number generation.
Explanation: Random number generation does not provide specific insights or details required for a rich, in-depth case study.

222. A limitation of using case studies in nursing leadership is:
a. The inability to generalize findings to broader populations.
b. The detailed information provided.
c. The focus on real-world problems.
d. The use of multiple data sources.


Answer: a. The inability to generalize findings to broader populations.
Explanation: Case studies offer deep insights into specific scenarios but may not always be generalizable to broader settings or groups.

223. To enhance the validity of a nursing leadership case study, a researcher should:
a. Focus only on positive outcomes.
b. Use a single data source for simplicity.
c. Incorporate multiple perspectives and data sources.
d. Make assumptions based on personal experience.


Answer: c. Incorporate multiple perspectives and data sources.
Explanation: Using multiple perspectives and data sources (triangulation) enriches the case study and adds validity to the findings.

224. When using a case study as a teaching tool, the nurse executive should encourage learners to:
a. Focus on memorizing the details of the case.
b. Provide answers as quickly as possible.
c. Reflect on and discuss the case's complexities.
d. Concentrate only on the final outcome of the case.


Answer: c. Reflect on and discuss the case's complexities.
Explanation: Discussion and reflection allow learners to analyze, understand, and internalize the intricacies of the case, fostering deeper learning.

225. Effective communication within a nursing unit is vital. Which of the following principles underpins the foundation of communication?
a. Using complex terminology to demonstrate expertise.
b. Delivering messages with consistency and clarity.
c. Avoiding feedback to maintain authority.
d. Communicating only when there's an issue.

Answer: b. Delivering messages with consistency and clarity.
Explanation: Effective communication requires that messages are clear and consistent to avoid misunderstandings and foster trust.

226. A nurse executive aims to improve interdisciplinary collaboration. What's the best strategy to encourage open communication among different departments?
a. Schedule regular interdepartmental meetings with a set agenda.
b. Encourage writing memos to document concerns.
c. Avoid discussing department-specific jargon in meetings.
d. Limit communication to only high-level executives.

Answer: a. Schedule regular interdepartmental meetings with a set agenda.
Explanation: Regular meetings with a clear agenda facilitate open communication, allowing for sharing insights and addressing concerns collaboratively.

227. Active listening is a cornerstone of effective communication. Which behavior exemplifies active listening?
a. Thinking about a response while the other person is speaking.
b. Frequently checking one's phone during a conversation.
c. Repeating back or paraphrasing what the speaker has said.
d. Advising the speaker without being asked for advice.

Answer: c. Repeating back or paraphrasing what the speaker has said.
Explanation: Active listening involves fully concentrating on, understanding, and responding to a speaker. Paraphrasing or repeating back validates understanding.

228. In relationship building, what should a nurse executive prioritize to foster trust within the team?
a. Ensuring team members only see the executive's strengths.
b. Avoiding challenging situations.
c. Being transparent, especially during difficult times.
d. Keeping personal and professional lives entirely separate.

Answer: c. Being transparent, especially during difficult times.
Explanation: Transparency, especially during challenges, builds trust as team members feel informed and valued.

229. Which communication channel is most suitable for discussing sensitive or complex issues with a nursing team member?
a. Email.
b. A group chat platform.
c. Face-to-face conversation.
d. Anonymous feedback box.

Answer: c. Face-to-face conversation.
Explanation: Face-to-face conversations are ideal for sensitive topics as they allow for immediate feedback, non-verbal cues, and a personal touch.

230. A nurse executive recognizes a gap in cultural competence within the team. Which strategy promotes understanding and effective communication across diverse cultures?
a. Avoid discussing cultural differences to prevent discomfort.
b. Organize training sessions on cultural competence.
c. Assume that all team members have the same cultural knowledge.
d. Encourage team members to only speak English, regardless of their native language.

Answer: b. Organize training sessions on cultural competence.
Explanation: Training sessions foster awareness, understanding, and skills to communicate effectively across diverse cultures.

231. A nurse executive is trying to build stronger relationships with team members. Which action can hinder relationship building?
a. Taking time to understand team members' personal goals.
b. Providing constructive feedback in a respectful manner.
c. Frequently canceling scheduled one-on-one meetings.
d. Acknowledging team members' achievements.

Answer: c. Frequently canceling scheduled one-on-one meetings.
Explanation: Consistency in engagement is crucial. Canceling meetings often may signal a lack of respect for others' time or lack of commitment.

232. For effective communication, how should a nurse executive approach delivering negative feedback?
a. Publicly, so others can learn from the example.
b. Vaguely, to avoid hurt feelings.
c. Directly and constructively, focusing on behaviors and not personality.
d. Through written communication only.

Answer: c. Directly and constructively, focusing on behaviors and not personality.
Explanation: Negative feedback is most effective when it's specific, focuses on behaviors (not personal attributes), and is delivered in a constructive manner.

233. A nurse executive wishes to foster a culture where team members feel free to share their insights. Which strategy supports this?
a. Creating a strict hierarchy of communication.
b. Encouraging an open-door policy.
c. Penalizing those who voice dissenting opinions.
d. Reserving communication for formal settings only.

Answer: b. Encouraging an open-door policy.
Explanation: An open-door policy promotes open communication, making team members feel their input is valued and considered.

234. Which action by a nurse executive best demonstrates the importance of relationship building in leadership?
a. Keeping a distance from team members to maintain authority.
b. Actively seeking input and feedback from team members.
c. Making decisions unilaterally without team involvement.
d. Encouraging competition among team members.

Answer: b. Actively seeking input and feedback from team members.
Explanation: Seeking input shows team members that their expertise is valued, fostering mutual respect and trust.

235. The Transactional Model of Communication considers which of the following as pivotal for effective communication?
a. The sender only.
b. The message content solely.
c. Both the sender and the receiver, emphasizing feedback.
d. The channel or medium used for communication.

Answer: c. Both the sender and the receiver, emphasizing feedback.
Explanation: The Transactional Model recognizes both the sender and receiver as active participants, highlighting the continuous feedback loop between them.

236. Active listening differs from passive listening in that active listening:
a. Consists of merely hearing words.
b. Involves interpreting and understanding the speaker's message.
c. Requires minimal feedback to the speaker.
d. Focuses only on the non-verbal cues of the speaker.


Answer: b. Involves interpreting and understanding the speaker's message.
Explanation: Active listening encompasses a deeper engagement with the speaker by understanding, interpreting, and responding to their message.

237. The Shannon-Weaver Model identifies noise as an external factor that can impede communication. In a healthcare setting, which of the following can be a source of "noise"?
a. Lack of medical terminology knowledge.
b. Effective electronic health record systems.
c. Regular team meetings.
d. Patient satisfaction.


Answer: a. Lack of medical terminology knowledge.
Explanation: In the context of the model, "noise" refers to any disruption that affects the clarity of the message. A lack of understanding of medical terminology can distort message interpretation.

238. Which technique is effective in ensuring that a message has been understood as intended in a healthcare setting?
a. Speaking louder.
b. Using only written communication.
c. Employing the "teach-back" method.
d. Using more medical jargon.


Answer: c. Employing the "teach-back" method.
Explanation: The "teach-back" method involves asking individuals to explain the information just provided, ensuring understanding and clarity.

239. Which of the following communication tools is essential in maintaining continuity of care in healthcare settings?
a. Casual chats among healthcare workers.
b. Social media platforms.
c. SBAR (Situation, Background, Assessment, Recommendation).
d. Informal notes.

Answer: c. SBAR (Situation, Background, Assessment, Recommendation).
Explanation: SBAR is a structured communication tool that ensures concise, relevant, and clear information exchange, vital for patient safety and care continuity.

240. The "feedback loop" in communication theories refers to:
a. Providing positive comments only.
b. The receiver's response or reaction to the message.
c. The original message from the sender.
d. The medium or channel of communication.

Answer: b. The receiver's response or reaction to the message. Explanation: The feedback loop encompasses the receiver's response, ensuring the sender understands how their message was perceived.

241. To ensure active listening, a nurse executive should prioritize:
a. Interrupting to provide solutions.
b. Mentally preparing a response while the other speaks.
c. Summarizing or paraphrasing the speaker's message.
d. Relying solely on written notes.

Answer: c. Summarizing or paraphrasing the speaker's message. Explanation: Paraphrasing or summarizing confirms understanding and demonstrates to the speaker that they have been genuinely heard.

242. Which of the following best defines the concept of "encoding" in communication theories?
a. The medium chosen for communication.
b. The process of interpreting a received message.
c. The conversion of thoughts into a communicable message.
d. External factors disrupting communication.

Answer: c. The conversion of thoughts into a communicable message.
Explanation: Encoding refers to the process where the sender transforms their thoughts or ideas into a message suitable for communication.

243. In a high-stress healthcare situation, which communication technique can be most effective?
a. Employing multiple communication channels simultaneously.
b. Using closed-ended questions for clarity and brevity.
c. Speaking rapidly to convey urgency.
d. Relying on non-verbal cues only.

Answer: b. Using closed-ended questions for clarity and brevity.
Explanation: In high-stress situations, clear and concise communication is crucial. Closed-ended questions can obtain specific information quickly.

244. To improve interdisciplinary communication in a healthcare setting, which of the following strategies can be employed?
a. Implementing a top-down communication approach.
b. Reducing the frequency of team meetings to avoid information overload.
c. Promoting a shared language or common terminology.
d. Encouraging departments to work in silos.

Answer: c. Promoting a shared language or common terminology.
Explanation: A shared language ensures that terms and phrases have a consistent meaning across disciplines, reducing misunderstandings.

245. In building a therapeutic relationship, it's crucial to recognize that:
a. Nurses should become friends with the patient.
b. The relationship is patient-centered.
c. The relationship is primarily built on mutual personal interests.
d. Keeping professional boundaries can hinder trust.

Answer: b. The relationship is patient-centered.
Explanation: A therapeutic relationship places the needs, feelings, and well-being of the patient at the forefront, ensuring the best possible care.

246. The Peplau's Nurse-Patient Relationship theory identifies different phases. Which phase involves the nurse aiding the patient in recognizing their feelings and exploring dysfunctions?
a. Orientation phase
b. Identification phase
c. Exploitation phase
d. Resolution phase

Answer: b. Identification phase
Explanation: In the identification phase, patients begin to voice feelings and explore problematic areas, with the nurse aiding in their recognition.

247. Which of the following is NOT an aspect of effective relationship management in a healthcare setting?
a. Clear communication
b. Assertive dominance
c. Mutual respect
d. Active listening

Answer: b. Assertive dominance
Explanation: Relationship management is about mutual respect, understanding, and collaboration. Dominating the relationship can hinder effective communication and trust.

248. For nurse executives, which skill is particularly vital in managing relationships among interdisciplinary teams?
a. Delivering top-down directives efficiently
b. Encouraging siloed department functioning
c. Emphasizing open communication and feedback
d. Focusing solely on the nursing department's concerns

Answer: c. Emphasizing open communication and feedback
Explanation: Open communication allows for better understanding, collaboration, and shared objectives among interdisciplinary teams.

249. Building therapeutic relationships is vital in nursing because:
a. It ensures the nurse is well-liked by the patient.
b. It guarantees patient compliance.
c. It facilitates better patient outcomes and experience.
d. It ensures the nurse's opinions are prioritized.

Answer: c. It facilitates better patient outcomes and experience.
Explanation: A strong therapeutic relationship fosters trust, effective communication, and a conducive environment for healing, leading to better outcomes.

250. A nurse executive learns of conflicts between nursing teams. Which approach reflects effective relationship management?
a. Implementing immediate disciplinary action without investigations
b. Taking sides based on personal relationships
c. Mediating discussions and encouraging open dialogue
d. Ignoring the conflict, hoping it resolves independently


Answer: c. Mediating discussions and encouraging open dialogue
Explanation: Addressing conflicts by facilitating open discussions helps in understanding concerns, fostering collaboration, and promoting resolution.

251. What is a potential barrier to building a therapeutic relationship in nursing?
a. Spending excessive time with one patient
b. Acknowledging a patient's emotions
c. Keeping professional boundaries
d. Showing empathy


Answer: a. Spending excessive time with one patient
Explanation: Allocating disproportionate time to one patient may neglect others' needs and blur professional boundaries.

252. For nurse executives managing relationships within their teams, which is an effective strategy for resolving interpersonal conflicts?
a. Encourage the involved parties to deal with it on their own.
b. Favor the senior staff member in disputes.
c. Facilitate a structured conflict resolution session.
d. Immediately reassign one of the conflicting members.


Answer: c. Facilitate a structured conflict resolution session.
Explanation: Addressing conflicts through structured sessions fosters understanding, mutual respect, and possible resolution.

253. A key element in building and sustaining therapeutic relationships is:
a. Offering personal contact details for any needed support.
b. Providing solutions without exploring the patient's feelings.
c. Demonstrating genuine concern and understanding.
d. Encouraging the patient to depend on the nurse for emotional support.

Answer: c. Demonstrating genuine concern and understanding.
Explanation: Genuine concern promotes trust, making the patient feel valued and understood, crucial for a therapeutic relationship.

254. In relationship management, a nurse executive should prioritize:
a. Building alliances based on personal friendships.
b. Ensuring that their decisions are unquestioned.
c. Promoting an environment of mutual trust and respect.
d. Keeping a strict professional distance from all staff.

Answer: c. Promoting an environment of mutual trust and respect.
Explanation: Mutual trust and respect are foundational for effective relationship management, fostering collaboration, and understanding.

255. Effective interdisciplinary collaboration is MOST closely associated with which of the following outcomes in patient care?
a. Decreased hospital readmissions
b. Increased individual department autonomy
c. Fragmented care delivery
d. Longer hospital stays

Answer: a. Decreased hospital readmissions
Explanation: Effective interdisciplinary collaboration ensures a comprehensive and cohesive approach to patient care, potentially reducing hospital readmissions due to more holistic care.

256. A primary goal of interdisciplinary collaboration in healthcare is to:
a. Ensure each department operates independently.
b. Maximize the dominance of a single profession.
c. Promote shared decision-making based on expertise.
d. Minimize input from auxiliary services.

Answer: c. Promote shared decision-making based on expertise.
Explanation: Interdisciplinary collaboration allows for pooling expertise from various professionals, ensuring decisions made are holistic and informed.

257. Which of the following strategies is LEAST effective for promoting interdisciplinary collaboration?
a. Ensuring clear communication among team members
b. Encouraging departmental silos
c. Offering interdisciplinary training sessions
d. Incorporating input from all relevant professions in care planning

Answer: b. Encouraging departmental silos
Explanation: Departmental silos restrict communication and collaboration between departments, counteracting interdisciplinary collaboration's goals.

258. Conflict within interdisciplinary teams can arise due to:
a. Uniform understanding of patient care goals
b. Overlapping scopes of practice
c. A shared vision for patient outcomes
d. Consistent communication patterns

Answer: b. Overlapping scopes of practice
Explanation: Overlapping roles can create confusion about responsibilities, leading to potential conflicts in decision-making or care provision.

259. To address conflicts in interdisciplinary teams effectively, nurse executives should:
a. Allow teams to resolve issues without any oversight.
b. Mandate unilateral decisions without team input.
c. Promote an open environment for voicing concerns.
d. Foster a competition-based approach to problem-solving.

Answer: c. Promote an open environment for voicing concerns.
Explanation: An open environment facilitates communication and understanding, allowing teams to address and resolve conflicts collaboratively.

260. A barrier to effective interdisciplinary collaboration can be:
a. Regular interdisciplinary team meetings
b. Clearly defined roles for each team member
c. Hierarchy-driven decision-making processes
d. Mutual respect for the expertise of each profession

Answer: c. Hierarchy-driven decision-making processes. Explanation: Hierarchical structures can limit the input of some team members, reducing the richness of interdisciplinary insights and potentially causing conflicts.

261. In the context of addressing conflict, active listening involves:
a. Waiting for your turn to respond while someone speaks.
b. Formulating counterarguments during discussions.
c. Truly understanding and considering the speaker's perspective.
d. Listening for gaps in arguments to identify weaknesses.

Answer: c. Truly understanding and considering the speaker's perspective.
Explanation: Active listening is about genuinely trying to understand the speaker's viewpoint, feelings, and concerns, promoting empathy and understanding.

262. Which technique is MOST effective for conflict resolution in interdisciplinary teams?
a. Avoiding conflict until it resolves itself
b. Addressing the issue directly with open dialogue
c. Implementing decisions without team consensus
d. Encouraging team members to address conflicts privately, away from the team

Answer: b. Addressing the issue directly with open dialogue. Explanation: Open dialogue ensures that all concerns are aired, discussed, and collaboratively addressed, promoting understanding and team cohesion.

263. A challenge in interdisciplinary collaboration in healthcare is:
a. Common language across professions
b. Different professional cultures and values
c. Unified treatment goals for patients
d. Shared decision-making mechanisms

Answer: b. Different professional cultures and values. Explanation: Different professions may have distinct cultures, values, and approaches, which can be a challenge in creating a cohesive collaborative environment.

264. When conflicts arise due to misunderstandings in interdisciplinary teams, nurse executives should FIRST:
a. Assign blame to the responsible party
b. Facilitate a team meeting for open communication
c. Transfer conflicting members to other teams
d. Ignore the issue, assuming professionals will resolve it themselves

Answer: b. Facilitate a team meeting for open communication
Explanation: Addressing misunderstandings promptly through open communication prevents escalation and fosters mutual understanding and respect.

265. Diversity in nursing involves considering:
a. Only the ethnic and cultural backgrounds of patients.
b. Only the ethnic and cultural backgrounds of nurses.
c. The varied backgrounds, experiences, and perspectives of both patients and nurses.
d. Only differences in age and gender of nurses.

Answer: c. The varied backgrounds, experiences, and perspectives of both patients and nurses.
Explanation: Diversity encompasses a wide range of differences, including but not limited to race, ethnicity, gender, age, physical abilities, etc., among both patients and healthcare providers.

266. When aiming for inclusivity in nursing practice, a primary objective is:
a. Making sure everyone speaks the same language.
b. Avoiding discussions about differences to prevent conflict.
c. Ensuring every patient and staff member feels valued, heard, and understood.
d. Standardizing care practices to treat everyone the same.

Answer: c. Ensuring every patient and staff member feels valued, heard, and understood.
Explanation: Inclusivity seeks to create environments where each individual feels they have a place and are understood and respected in their entirety.

267. To celebrate diversity in a nursing unit, nurse leaders can:
a. Make sure everyone conforms to a single culture for unity.
b. Organize events that recognize and appreciate various cultural traditions.
c. Encourage staff to keep personal cultural practices private.
d. Implement a one-size-fits-all approach to patient care.

Answer: b. Organize events that recognize and appreciate various cultural traditions.
Explanation: Celebrating diversity means acknowledging and valuing differences. By organizing events that appreciate various traditions, nurse leaders can create an inclusive environment.

268. A strategy to promote inclusivity in nursing practice is:
a. Providing care based on assumptions.
b. Actively seeking feedback from diverse team members and patients.
c. Ensuring all staff members have identical viewpoints.
d. Avoiding discussions about race and ethnicity.

Answer: b. Actively seeking feedback from diverse team members and patients.
Explanation: Actively seeking feedback ensures that all voices are heard, fostering an environment where diverse perspectives are valued and included.

269. Which of the following is an advantage of having a diverse nursing team?
a. Easier management due to homogeneity.
b. Enhanced patient trust and rapport through representation.
c. Reduced need for cultural competency training.
d. Elimination of potential conflicts in the team.

Answer: b. Enhanced patient trust and rapport through representation.
Explanation: When patients see themselves represented within the care team, it can foster a sense of understanding and trust.

270. In addressing unconscious bias in nursing, it is important to:
a. Assume it doesn't exist unless proven.
b. Recognize and confront it through training and self-awareness.
c. Consider it only as an external issue.
d. Rely solely on personal experiences to shape care decisions.

Answer: b. Recognize and confront it through training and self-awareness.
Explanation: Unconscious bias affects everyone. Recognizing its existence and actively working to mitigate its effects is crucial in inclusive nursing practice.

271. A common barrier to inclusivity in nursing is:
a. Overemphasis on cultural competency.
b. A diverse patient demographic.
c. Stereotyping and assumptions.
d. Regular team discussions on diversity.

Answer: c. Stereotyping and assumptions.
Explanation: Stereotyping and making assumptions about individuals based on perceived group affiliations can hinder genuine understanding and inclusivity.

272. A nurse executive promoting inclusivity should:
a. Implement policies without seeking diverse perspectives.
b. Only consider input from senior nurses.
c. Engage in active listening when staff or patients express concerns.
d. Discourage team members from sharing their cultural backgrounds.

Answer: c. Engage in active listening when staff or patients express concerns.
Explanation: Active listening is fundamental in understanding and addressing concerns related to diversity and inclusivity.

273. The ultimate goal of inclusive nursing practice is to:
a. Simplify administrative processes.
b. Ensure every individual receives equitable, personalized care.
c. Reduce the need for diverse hiring.
d. Limit patient-nurse interactions to clinical discussions.

Answer: b. Ensure every individual receives equitable, personalized care.
Explanation: The heart of inclusivity in nursing is providing care that recognizes and addresses individual needs, backgrounds, and perspectives.

274. In fostering an inclusive environment, nurse executives should:
a. Emphasize conformity to a single standard.
b. Encourage open dialogue about diversity and its challenges.
c. Hire staff based solely on cultural background.
d. Limit patient feedback to clinical outcomes.

Answer: b. Encourage open dialogue about diversity and its challenges.
Explanation: Open dialogue can lead to a better understanding of challenges and facilitate collaborative solutions to address them, thereby fostering inclusivity.

275. The core principle of patient-centered care is:
a. Focusing only on the disease process.
b. Implementing standardized care for all patients.
c. Partnering with patients in their care decisions.
d. Relying on the physician's decisions for patient outcomes.

Answer: c. Partnering with patients in their care decisions.
Explanation: Patient-centered care emphasizes the importance of the patient's perspective, needs, and preferences in the decision-making process.

276. Which of the following models of care emphasizes the role of a nurse as a primary care coordinator, delegating tasks to auxiliary staff?
a. Total Patient Care
b. Team Nursing
c. Case Method Nursing
d. Functional Nursing

Answer: b. Team Nursing
Explanation: In team nursing, a registered nurse leads nursing personnel (LPNs, CNAs) to deliver patient care as a team.

277. In the Total Patient Care model, responsibility for care primarily rests with:
a. A designated physician.
b. A team of varied professionals.
c. An individual nurse.
d. Auxiliary staff.

Answer: c. An individual nurse.
Explanation: In the Total Patient Care model, also known as the Case Method, one nurse is responsible for all aspects of care for one or more patients.

278. One potential drawback of the Functional Nursing model is:
a. Limited individual accountability.
b. Overemphasis on the patient's perspective.
c. Too much reliance on one nurse.
d. A lack of delegation.

Answer: a. Limited individual accountability.
Explanation: In Functional Nursing, tasks are divided among staff members based on their function, which can sometimes lead to fragmented care and reduced accountability.

279. The nursing model that promotes a holistic approach, focusing on the interconnectedness of physical, psychological, social, and spiritual needs is:
a. Biomedical Model
b. Integrative Care
c. Functional Nursing
d. Primary Nursing

Answer: b. Integrative Care
Explanation: Integrative care focuses on the whole person, emphasizing the connection between mind, body, and spirit, and often incorporates complementary therapies.

280. A key advantage of Team Nursing is:
a. Reduction in the skill mix of the team.
b. Focusing only on specific tasks.
c. Efficient use of varied expertise within a team.
d. Elimination of the role of the primary nurse.

Answer: c. Efficient use of varied expertise within a team.
Explanation: Team nursing capitalizes on the diverse skills of each team member, allowing for efficient and comprehensive care.

281. The core principle of Primary Nursing is:
a. Delegating most tasks to other team members.
b. One nurse being responsible for total care during their working hours.
c. Dividing tasks based on function.
d. Ignoring the patient's preferences.

Answer: b. One nurse being responsible for total care during their working hours.
Explanation: In Primary Nursing, one nurse maintains responsibility for the care of a patient throughout their stay.

282. In considering models of care, a Nurse Executive must:
a. Implement the latest model without evaluation.
b. Only consider cost-effectiveness.
c. Ensure alignment with the institution's mission and patient population needs.
d. Avoid including frontline staff in the decision-making process.

Answer: c. Ensure alignment with the institution's mission and patient population needs.
Explanation: The most effective model of care is contingent on the specific needs of the patient population and the overall mission and values of the healthcare institution.

283. Patient-centered care emphasizes:
a. Sole reliance on clinical evidence for decision-making.
b. A passive role for patients in their care.
c. Collaborative partnerships with families and caregivers.
d. Limiting options based on institutional preferences.

Answer: c. Collaborative partnerships with families and caregivers.
Explanation: Patient-centered care focuses on forming partnerships with patients and their families to ensure care decisions align with their desires and values.

284. Which model of care allows a nurse to follow a patient across various care settings, ensuring continuity of care?
a. Total Patient Care
b. Case Management
c. Team Nursing
d. Functional Nursing

Answer: b. Case Management. Explanation: The Case Management model focuses on coordinating and streamlining services for specific patient populations across different settings, ensuring continuity and optimizing patient outcomes.

285. Which of the following is a primary goal of care coordination?
a. Ensuring patients see as many specialists as possible.
b. Reducing healthcare costs without regard for outcome.
c. Facilitating the appropriate delivery of healthcare services.
d. Limiting patient choice in healthcare decisions.

Answer: c. Facilitating the appropriate delivery of healthcare services. Explanation: Care coordination seeks to organize and facilitate patient care to ensure they receive the right services at the right time.

286. One of the key risks associated with poor transition of care is:
a. Reduced hospital admissions.
b. Enhanced patient satisfaction.
c. Medication errors.
d. Improved communication among care teams.


Answer: c. Medication errors.
Explanation: Inadequate transitions of care can lead to oversight and miscommunication, which can result in medication errors.

287. A key strategy for effective transition of care is:
a. Ignoring patient and family preferences.
b. Ensuring discharge summaries are communicated to the next provider of care.
c. Limiting information to reduce confusion.
d. Discouraging patients from asking questions about their care.


Answer: b. Ensuring discharge summaries are communicated to the next provider of care.
Explanation: Communication between providers ensures that the receiving provider is aware of the patient's status, ongoing needs, and any potential concerns.

288. The Interprofessional Care Plan is a tool that:
a. Dictates a prescriptive approach to patient care without flexibility.
b. Is solely for the nursing team to review and update.
c. Encourages siloed care without team input.
d. Facilitates a collaborative approach to patient-centered care.


Answer: d. Facilitates a collaborative approach to patient-centered care.
Explanation: Interprofessional Care Plans are designed to be collaborative tools that encompass input from various care team members, ensuring comprehensive and patient-centered care.

289. In care coordination, the use of electronic health records (EHR) primarily benefits by:
a. Increasing the redundancy of medical tests.
b. Facilitating communication and information sharing among healthcare professionals.
c. Discouraging patient engagement in their care.
d. Limiting access to patient health information.

Answer: b. Facilitating communication and information sharing among healthcare professionals.
Explanation: EHR systems enable seamless sharing of patient information across providers and institutions, ensuring coordinated and informed care.

290. A primary challenge in transitions of care for chronic disease patients is:
a. Limited patient involvement in acute settings.
b. Simplistic care plans.
c. Gaps in communication and potential for fragmented care.
d. Overcommunication between healthcare providers.

Answer: c. Gaps in communication and potential for fragmented care.
Explanation: Chronic disease patients often engage with multiple healthcare providers across various settings. Without effective transition processes, there's potential for communication breakdowns and fragmented care.

291. Which of the following is NOT typically a role of a care coordinator?
a. Assisting patients in understanding their care plans.
b. Ordering medications without consulting a physician.
c. Facilitating communication between healthcare providers.
d. Advocating for patients' needs and preferences.

Answer: b. Ordering medications without consulting a physician.
Explanation: Care coordinators are primarily responsible for facilitating care and ensuring smooth transitions, not for making independent medical decisions such as medication orders.

292. For a patient transitioning from acute care to home care, which tool would be essential for ensuring continuity of care?
a. A brochure of the hospital's achievements.
b. A list of local pharmacies.
c. Detailed discharge instructions and a care plan.
d. The contact information of all staff who cared for the patient during their hospital stay.

Answer: c. Detailed discharge instructions and a care plan.
Explanation: To ensure continuity of care, patients and caregivers need comprehensive instructions and care plans that guide their next steps in the care journey.

293. One of the main reasons for readmission after discharge is:
a. Too much patient autonomy.
b. Overly detailed discharge instructions.
c. Inadequate follow-up care and understanding of post-discharge needs.
d. Prolonged initial hospital stays.


Answer: c. Inadequate follow-up care and understanding of post-discharge needs.
Explanation: A significant factor in readmissions is the gap in follow-up care and a lack of understanding or resources to manage post-discharge needs.

294. A crucial step in ensuring effective care coordination is:
a. Avoiding over-reliance on technology.
b. Implementing strategies without patient feedback.
c. Fostering open communication and trust among interdisciplinary team members.
d. Keeping care plans static regardless of changing patient needs.


Answer: c. Fostering open communication and trust among interdisciplinary team members.
Explanation: Trust and open lines of communication among team members are fundamental for coordinating care effectively, ensuring everyone is on the same page and working toward unified patient goals.

295. In the realm of quality improvement, the acronym PDSA stands for:
a. Problem, Direction, Solution, Assessment
b. Plan, Do, Study, Act
c. Process, Deliver, Secure, Achieve
d. Patient, Doctor, Service, Admin


Answer: b. Plan, Do, Study, Act
Explanation: The PDSA cycle is a fundamental QI tool that involves planning a change, implementing the change, studying the results, and determining what modifications are necessary.

296. The primary goal of Quality Improvement in nursing is:
a. Reducing the cost of healthcare services.
b. Eliminating the need for interdisciplinary collaboration.
c. Continually advancing the quality of patient care.
d. Documenting errors without any follow-up action.

Answer: c. Continually advancing the quality of patient care.
Explanation: Quality Improvement aims to enhance the level of patient care and outcomes continuously by analyzing current processes and making necessary changes.

297. Which of the following is NOT a standard tool used in QI processes?
a. Fishbone diagram
b. SWOT analysis
c. Histogram
d. PESTLE analysis

Answer: d. PESTLE analysis
Explanation: PESTLE (Political, Economic, Sociocultural, Technological, Legal, Environmental) analysis is more commonly used for strategic management, not specific to QI processes in nursing.

298. addressing this through a QI process is:
a. Assign blame to the nursing staff.
b. Introduce a new policy immediately.
c. Conduct a root cause analysis.
d. Disregard the increase as a random event.

Answer: c. Conduct a root cause analysis. Explanation: A root cause analysis is used to determine the underlying reasons for a problem, making it a fundamental first step in the QI process.

299. The Pareto Chart in QI processes helps in:
a. Identifying the most frequent causes of a problem.
b. Displaying data in chronological order.
c. Tracking individual patient health metrics.
d. Comparing two unrelated problems in a healthcare setting.

Answer: a. Identifying the most frequent causes of a problem.
Explanation: The Pareto Chart, or the "80/20 rule," helps identify the major causes of a problem, allowing teams to focus their improvement efforts effectively.

300. Which statement best defines the "Six Sigma" approach to QI?
a. A focus on team communication only.
b. A process that strives for near-perfect results.
c. A method that disregards statistical analysis.
d. An approach that accepts a certain level of errors as unavoidable.

Answer: b. A process that strives for near-perfect results.
Explanation: Six Sigma is a QI methodology that seeks to reduce defects and improve processes to achieve near-perfect (99.99966%) outcomes.

301. Run charts are essential in QI for:
a. Establishing a cause-and-effect relationship with certainty.
b. Displaying qualitative data only.
c. Observing data over time and identifying trends.
d. Setting the annual budget for a nursing unit.

Answer: c. Observing data over time and identifying trends.
Explanation: Run charts are visual tools that display data points over time, helping in the identification of trends, shifts, or cycles.

302. Control charts differ from run charts because they:
a. Display data over time.
b. Ignore variations in data.
c. Incorporate upper and lower control limits.
d. Only focus on financial metrics.

Answer: c. Incorporate upper and lower control limits.
Explanation: While both control and run charts display data over time, control charts also establish control limits to distinguish between common-cause and special-cause variations.

303. Continuous Quality Improvement (CQI) in nursing is best described as:
a. A short-term approach to solving immediate problems.
b. A process that focuses only on large-scale issues.
c. An ongoing effort to improve the quality of patient care.
d. An approach that emphasizes punitive measures for mistakes.

Answer: c. An ongoing effort to improve the quality of patient care.
Explanation: CQI is a philosophy that emphasizes the continuous efforts of healthcare professionals to enhance patient care by constantly assessing and improving processes.

304. One of the main benefits of using Quality Improvement tools in nursing is:
a. Reinforcing hierarchical structures in a team.
b. Addressing only externally reported problems.
c. Bypassing the need for evidence-based practices.
d. Identifying inefficiencies and areas for improvement in care processes.

Answer: d. Identifying inefficiencies and areas for improvement in care processes.
Explanation: QI tools and methodologies aid in uncovering areas where processes can be enhanced, ensuring the delivery of optimal patient care.

305. One of the primary purposes of regulatory compliance in healthcare is to:
a. Increase the financial profitability of the healthcare institution.
b. Decrease the reliance on interdisciplinary collaboration.
c. Ensure patient safety and enhance the quality of care.
d. Limit the need for advanced medical technology in patient care.

Answer: c. Ensure patient safety and enhance the quality of care.
Explanation: Regulatory compliance primarily aims to uphold standards that safeguard patient well-being and elevate the quality of healthcare services.

306. Which regulatory body sets standards for the privacy and security of patient health information?
a. Occupational Safety and Health Administration (OSHA)
b. Joint Commission
c. Centers for Medicare & Medicaid Services (CMS)
d. Health Insurance Portability and Accountability Act (HIPAA)

Answer: d. Health Insurance Portability and Accountability Act (HIPAA)
Explanation: HIPAA establishes national standards for the privacy and security of patient health information, ensuring patient confidentiality.

307. When preparing for an accreditation visit from the Joint Commission, a nurse executive should prioritize:
a. Halting all patient care services to focus solely on the accreditation.
b. Creating a one-time event to quickly train all staff members.
c. Establishing a continuous culture of compliance and readiness.
d. Only preparing those departments that had issues during the last audit.

Answer: c. Establishing a continuous culture of compliance and readiness.
Explanation: Continuously promoting a culture of readiness ensures that the organization is always prepared for accreditation reviews, not just during the audit period.

308. An unexpected survey visit from a regulatory or accrediting body is often referred to as a:
a. Planned assessment.
b. Spot check.
c. Proactive review.
d. Surprise survey.

Answer: b. Spot check.
Explanation: A spot check or unannounced survey ensures that organizations maintain compliance consistently, not just during scheduled reviews.

309. Which of the following is a PRIMARY reason why healthcare institutions seek accreditation from bodies like the Joint Commission?
a. To gain a competitive edge in marketing.
b. To reduce the need for internal quality assurance processes.
c. To validate the quality and safety of the care they provide.
d. To ensure higher salaries for their healthcare professionals.

Answer: c. To validate the quality and safety of the care they provide.
Explanation: Accreditation from reputable bodies validates an institution's commitment to maintaining high-quality and safety standards in patient care.

310. To ensure preparedness for audits, an efficient strategy for a nurse executive would be:
a. Maintain up-to-date documentation and regular self-assessments.
b. Reactively address only those areas that were problematic in the past.
c. Limit staff involvement and delegate all tasks to a single department.
d. Avoid using technology or digital platforms for record-keeping.

Answer: a. Maintain up-to-date documentation and regular self-assessments.
Explanation: Regularly updating documentation and conducting internal assessments ensures continuous compliance and readiness for external audits.

311. When a healthcare organization fails to meet a specific standard during an accreditation visit, this is usually termed as a:
a. Recommendation.
b. Deficiency.
c. Suggestion.
d. Guideline violation.

Answer: b. Deficiency.
Explanation: Deficiencies indicate that a particular standard or requirement set by the accrediting body has not been met by the healthcare organization.

312. Which entity is primarily responsible for regulating the participation of healthcare organizations in the Medicare and Medicaid programs?
a. American Nursing Association (ANA)
b. The World Health Organization (WHO)
c. The Joint Commission
d. Centers for Medicare & Medicaid Services (CMS)

Answer: d. Centers for Medicare & Medicaid Services (CMS)
Explanation: CMS oversees the federal Medicare program and collaborates with states on the Medicaid program, setting regulations for participation.

313. The use of evidence-based practice in nursing care:
a. Decreases the chances of regulatory compliance.
b. Is discouraged by most accreditation bodies.
c. Supports adherence to best practice standards set by regulatory bodies.
d. Is unrelated to regulatory and accreditation standards.

Answer: c. Supports adherence to best practice standards set by regulatory bodies.
Explanation: Using evidence-based practices aligns nursing care with the latest research and best practices, aiding in meeting or exceeding regulatory standards.

314. To ensure compliance with set standards, nurse executives should promote:
a. A culture that hides mistakes to avoid penalties.
b. An environment of continuous learning and improvement.
c. A focus solely on external audits and ignore internal assessments.
d. Decisions made without interdisciplinary collaborations.

Answer: b. An environment of continuous learning and improvement.
Explanation: Fostering a culture of continuous learning and enhancement ensures that care standards are consistently met and even exceeded.

315. In healthcare economics, the concept that healthcare resources are limited, and choices must be made about their allocation is termed:
a. Health determinism.
b. Resource stagnation.
c. Economic precision.
d. Scarcity.

Answer: d. Scarcity.
Explanation: Scarcity acknowledges that resources in healthcare are finite, emphasizing the need for judicious use and allocation decisions.

316. A nurse executive in a hospital is developing a budget for the upcoming year. Which of the following budgeting approaches bases the new budget on the actual performance of the current year, adjusting for future needs?
a. Zero-based budgeting.
b. Incremental budgeting.
c. Fixed budgeting.
d. Performance-based budgeting.

Answer: b. Incremental budgeting.
Explanation: Incremental budgeting takes into account the current year's performance and makes adjustments (increments) for the upcoming year based on anticipated needs.

317. In the context of reimbursement models, what does DRG stand for?
a. Directed Reimbursement Group.
b. Diagnostic Related Group.
c. Diverse Rate Group.
d. Direct Rate Generators.

Answer: b. Diagnostic Related Group.
Explanation: DRGs are used as a system to classify hospital cases into one of approximately 500 groups, expecting to have similar hospital resource use, used for reimbursement purposes.

318. Which financing model pays the healthcare provider a set amount for each enrolled person assigned to them, per period of time, regardless of whether that person seeks care?
a. Fee-for-service.
b. Capitation.
c. Value-based reimbursement.
d. Bundled payment.

Answer: b. Capitation.
Explanation: In a capitation payment system, a set amount is paid to the healthcare provider for each enrolled person, irrespective of whether they accessed services or not.

319. A nurse executive is evaluating two potential capital expenditures for a nursing unit. The method that assesses the potential returns of the investment relative to its cost is:
a. Zero-based assessment.
b. Return on Investment (ROI).
c. Direct costing.
d. Variable assessment.

Answer: b. Return on Investment (ROI).
Explanation: ROI is a performance measure used to evaluate the efficiency of an investment or compare the efficiency of several investments.

320. Which of the following reimbursement models emphasizes payments based on the quality and efficiency of the care provided?
a. Fee-for-service.
b. Capitation.
c. Value-based reimbursement.
d. Per diem payment system.

Answer: c. Value-based reimbursement.
Explanation: Value-based reimbursement models reward healthcare providers based on the quality and efficiency of care, moving away from volume-based models.

321. When considering healthcare costs from an economic standpoint, indirect costs refer to:
a. Charges directly linked to specific treatments or procedures.
b. Expenses associated with overhead and administration.
c. Costs not directly linked to medical services, such as lost productivity.
d. The sum total of all medical bills incurred by a patient.

Answer: c. Costs not directly linked to medical services, such as lost productivity.
Explanation: Indirect costs encompass non-medical costs that arise due to illness, such as lost wages, reduced productivity, or other opportunity costs.

322. For nurse executives, understanding the concept of "opportunity cost" is essential. This term refers to:
a. The cost associated with the next-best alternative foregone.
b. Costs directly incurred from selecting an option.
c. Costs only related to financial transactions.
d. The financial benefits gained from choosing an option.


Answer: a. The cost associated with the next-best alternative foregone.
Explanation: Opportunity cost relates to the benefits one could have received from the next best alternative when a decision is made.

323. In a fixed budget, the nurse executive understands that:
a. Expenditures and revenues adjust depending on volume.
b. Costs change, but revenue remains constant.
c. Budgeted amounts remain unchanged regardless of the volume of services.
d. Financial planning is unnecessary.


Answer: c. Budgeted amounts remain unchanged regardless of the volume of services.
Explanation: A fixed budget is set at one level of activity and is not adjusted for actual levels of patient volume or services provided.

324. Which of the following budgeting methodologies requires each department to justify every aspect of its budget from scratch, as if the programs were being newly launched?
a. Incremental budgeting.
b. Zero-based budgeting.
c. Fixed budgeting.
d. Performance-based budgeting.


Answer: b. Zero-based budgeting.
Explanation: Zero-based budgeting starts from "zero base" and every function within an organization is analyzed for its needs and costs, making it as if everything is new.

325. Which level of health policy primarily focuses on issues like city hospital regulations or local health department protocols?
a. National
b. State
c. Local
d. International

Answer: c. Local
Explanation: Local health policies primarily deal with city or county-level issues, which can encompass regulations related to city hospitals or protocols for local health departments.

326. A nurse executive seeks to influence the development of a state policy that would impact advanced practice nursing regulations. The most appropriate organization to join for this advocacy work would be:
a. The World Health Organization (WHO).
b. The local city council.
c. State Nurse Association.
d. The American Hospital Association.

Answer: c. State Nurse Association.
Explanation: State Nurse Associations represent nurses at the state level and often engage in advocacy work related to state regulations and policies impacting nursing.

327. The Patient Protection and Affordable Care Act (ACA) is an example of a health policy at which level?
a. Local
b. State
c. National
d. Hospital-based

Answer: c. National
Explanation: The ACA is a federal legislation, making it a national health policy affecting healthcare across the U.S.

328. When a nurse executive is considering the impact of health policies on nursing practice, it is essential to review:
a. Only the policies directly mentioning nursing.
b. All health policies, as they may have direct or indirect effects on nursing.
c. Only state and local policies.
d. Only policies related to nursing education.

Answer: b. All health policies, as they may have direct or indirect effects on nursing.
Explanation: Health policies, even if they don't directly mention nursing, can have a profound direct or indirect impact on nursing practice, patient care, and the overall healthcare system.

329. Which organization is primarily responsible for making recommendations on the amounts and types of services that Medicare should cover at the national level?
a. Centers for Medicare & Medicaid Services (CMS)
b. The American Nurses Association
c. The National Institutes of Health
d. The Health Resources and Services Administration

Answer: a. Centers for Medicare & Medicaid Services (CMS)
Explanation: CMS is the federal agency responsible for the administration of Medicare and makes determinations about service coverages.

330. A nurse executive is concerned about the rising incidence of a specific disease within their community. To influence local policy changes, the nurse executive should FIRST:
a. Publish an article in a medical journal.
b. Lobby at the national level.
c. Engage with local health departments and city councils.
d. Await for national policies to trickle down.

Answer: c. Engage with local health departments and city councils.
Explanation: For immediate and localized concerns, engaging directly with local health departments and city councils can be effective in influencing local health policies.

331. Which policy level would MOST likely address licensure requirements for nurses?
a. Local
b. State
c. National
d. Hospital-based

Answer: b. State
Explanation: State-level policies typically govern licensure requirements for healthcare professionals, including nurses.

332. In the context of health policies, the term "scope of practice" primarily relates to:
a. The geographical area where a nurse can practice.
b. The range of services nurses are competent and authorized to perform.
c. The number of patients a nurse can care for during a shift.
d. The type of medications a nurse can prescribe.

Answer: b. The range of services nurses are competent and authorized to perform.
Explanation: Scope of practice defines the procedures, actions, and processes that a healthcare practitioner is permitted to undertake based on their professional license.

333. A nurse executive is trying to address nurse staffing ratios in her hospital. While she can develop internal guidelines, legally mandated ratios would be determined by:
a. The American Nurses Association.
b. Individual hospital boards.
c. State legislation.
d. National Council of State Boards of Nursing.

Answer: c. State legislation.
Explanation: Legally mandated nurse staffing ratios, where they exist, are typically determined by state legislation.

334. A new national health policy is enacted. As a nurse executive, what is the FIRST step to ensure that the healthcare organization is compliant with this policy?
a. Implement the changes immediately without review.
b. Await for local policies to provide guidance.
c. Understand and review the policy, then develop an implementation strategy.
d. Ask the nursing staff about their opinions on the policy.

Answer: c. Understand and review the policy, then develop an implementation strategy.
Explanation: It's crucial to first understand and thoroughly review a new policy. Once its implications are clear, an informed strategy can be developed for implementation to ensure compliance.

335. Which healthcare delivery model focuses on a team of primary care and specialist providers collaborating to provide comprehensive care for patients with complex needs?
a. Fee-for-service model
b. Patient-centered medical home
c. Direct primary care
d. Managed care organization

Answer: b. Patient-centered medical home
Explanation: The patient-centered medical home is designed to offer comprehensive and coordinated care for patients, especially those with complex needs, with an emphasis on primary care and collaboration among providers.

336. In the capitated payment model, how is a healthcare provider reimbursed?
a. Based on the number of services provided
b. A flat rate per member per month, regardless of the services rendered
c. Based on the quality outcomes achieved for care provided
d. On the number of referrals made to specialists

Answer: b. A flat rate per member per month, regardless of the services rendered
Explanation: In capitated payment models, providers receive a set amount per enrolled member, whether or not that member seeks care.

337. Which healthcare delivery model primarily emphasizes prevention, early detection, and health education?
a. Acute care model
b. Tertiary care model
c. Preventive care model
d. Urgent care model

Answer: c. Preventive care model
Explanation: The preventive care model is designed to emphasize early detection, health education, and prevention of diseases rather than treatment after the fact.

338. How does the Accountable Care Organization (ACO) model aim to reduce healthcare costs?
a. By prioritizing acute care over preventive care
b. By charging patients more for out-of-network services
c. By coordinating care and meeting specific quality benchmarks
d. By limiting the number of specialists in their network

Answer: c. By coordinating care and meeting specific quality benchmarks
Explanation: ACOs are designed to improve care coordination, reduce duplication of services, and meet quality benchmarks, which can result in cost savings.

339. Which delivery model aims to address healthcare disparities in underserved rural or urban areas?
a. Concierge medicine
b. Community health center model
c. Private practice model
d. Telehealth services

Answer: b. Community health center model
Explanation: Community health centers are established in underserved areas to provide comprehensive healthcare services, thus aiming to reduce healthcare disparities.

340. In which healthcare delivery model are healthcare providers employees of the hospital and are salaried rather than reimbursed per service?
a. Managed care organization
b. Fee-for-service model
c. Group practice model
d. Staff model HMO

Answer: d. Staff model HMO
Explanation: In the staff model HMO, providers are salaried employees of the health maintenance organization and typically provide services within HMO-owned facilities.

341. The transition to value-based care from volume-based care primarily aims to:
a. Increase the quantity of care provided.
b. Reduce the number of specialists in the healthcare system.
c. Improve patient outcomes and care efficiency.
d. Streamline administrative processes only.

Answer: c. Improve patient outcomes and care efficiency.
Explanation: Value-based care focuses on improving the quality and outcome of care delivered, emphasizing patient outcomes and efficiency rather than the volume of services provided.

342. A nurse executive working in a healthcare system that focuses on global budgets should prioritize:
a. Offering as many services as possible regardless of patient outcomes.
b. Coordinating care to provide necessary services within a fixed annual budget.
c. Limiting access to care to reduce costs.
d. Ignoring preventive care to prioritize immediate patient needs.

Answer: b. Coordinating care to provide necessary services within a fixed annual budget.
Explanation: In a global budget system, healthcare providers have a fixed annual budget to care for their patient population, which necessitates careful coordination and management of resources.

343. Which of the following models primarily operates on a subscription-based method where patients pay a monthly or annual fee directly to the physician for enhanced care services?
a. Direct primary care
b. Fee-for-service model
c. Managed care organization
d. Patient-centered medical home

Answer: a. Direct primary care
Explanation: Direct primary care operates on a subscription basis where patients pay physicians directly (bypassing insurance), often resulting in more personalized care and longer appointment times.

344. In a healthcare delivery model that emphasizes integrated care, a nurse executive should focus on:
a. Working in silos to maximize departmental efficiency.
b. Focusing solely on nursing services and disregarding other health professionals.
c. Facilitating collaboration and communication across various healthcare disciplines.
d. Relying solely on external consultants for care integration strategies.

Answer: c. Facilitating collaboration and communication across various healthcare disciplines.
Explanation: Integrated care emphasizes the coordinated delivery of services across the healthcare spectrum, necessitating collaboration and communication across various healthcare disciplines.

345. In the context of strategic management in healthcare, which tool provides a snapshot of an organization's internal strengths, weaknesses and its external opportunities and threats?
a. PDSA Cycle
b. Fishbone Diagram
c. SWOT Analysis
d. Gantt Chart

Answer: c. SWOT Analysis
Explanation: SWOT Analysis evaluates Strengths, Weaknesses, Opportunities, and Threats. This tool provides a clear view of internal and external factors influencing an organization, crucial for strategic planning.

346. When beginning the strategic planning process, what should a nurse executive prioritize first?
a. Analyzing the finances of the organization
b. Setting long-term goals
c. Understanding the organization's current state and mission
d. Designing specific interventions

Answer: c. Understanding the organization's current state and mission
Explanation: A strategic plan must align with the organization's mission and current state. Recognizing where the organization currently stands is essential to plan for its future.

347. In implementing a new evidence-based protocol, what should a nurse executive first consider?
a. How competitors are implementing similar protocols
b. The budgetary constraints of the organization
c. The potential resistance from the nursing staff
d. The current standard of care and its outcomes

Answer: d. The current standard of care and its outcomes
Explanation: Understanding the current standard of care and its outcomes helps identify gaps and areas for improvement, justifying the need for change and establishing a baseline for measuring the new protocol's success.

348. Which of the following is crucial when evaluating the success of a strategic initiative?
a. Comparing the initiative to those in other industries
b. Using subjective feedback only
c. Aligning outcomes with set benchmarks and goals
d. Focusing solely on immediate short-term gains

Answer: c. Aligning outcomes with set benchmarks and goals
Explanation: To evaluate a strategic initiative's success, outcomes should be compared against predetermined benchmarks and goals to determine if the initiative is on track or requires adjustments.

349. For a strategic plan to be successfully implemented, what role should leadership play?
a. Dictating each step to staff
b. Being passive and waiting for results
c. Engaging and inspiring staff towards the vision
d. Delegating all responsibilities to middle management

Answer: c. Engaging and inspiring staff towards the vision

Explanation: Effective leadership engages and motivates the staff, creating a shared vision that facilitates buy-in and collective effort towards achieving strategic goals.

350. Which tool is most effective in visually tracking the progress of a project over time and determining if tasks are being completed as scheduled?
a. PDSA Cycle
b. Fishbone Diagram
c. SWOT Analysis
d. Gantt Chart

Answer: d. Gantt Chart

Explanation: A Gantt Chart provides a visual representation of a project's timeline, including start and end dates for tasks, helping managers track progress and ensure tasks are completed on schedule.

351. When encountering resistance to change in the strategic implementation process, what is a key strategy for a nurse executive?
a. Ignoring the resistance and pushing forward
b. Engaging stakeholders and addressing their concerns
c. Overhauling the entire plan based on minor feedback
d. Focusing solely on external stakeholders

Answer: b. Engaging stakeholders and addressing their concerns

Explanation: Engaging stakeholders and addressing their concerns fosters understanding, buy-in, and collaboration, crucial for successful change management.

352. In the context of feedback, which method is most useful for continuous improvement in healthcare settings?
a. Waiting for annual reviews to address issues
b. Implementing changes without any feedback
c. Using a cyclical, iterative process of Plan-Do-Study-Act
d. Relying solely on patient feedback for process improvement

Answer: c. Using a cyclical, iterative process of Plan-Do-Study-Act

Explanation: The Plan-Do-Study-Act (PDSA) cycle is an iterative process designed for continuous improvement, allowing for frequent evaluations and adjustments based on feedback.

353. Which approach ensures that a strategic plan remains relevant amidst rapidly changing healthcare environments?
a. Creating a fixed, unchangeable five-year plan
b. Ignoring emerging healthcare trends
c. Engaging in frequent reassessments and adaptability
d. Solely focusing on internal organizational metrics

Answer: c. Engaging in frequent reassessments and adaptability
Explanation: Given the dynamic nature of healthcare, frequent reassessments and adaptability ensure that strategic plans remain aligned with changing environments and emerging needs.

354. To ensure financial sustainability while implementing a strategic plan, a nurse executive should prioritize:
a. Cutting staff to save costs
b. Ignoring financial metrics and focusing solely on patient outcomes
c. Aligning resource allocation with strategic priorities
d. Avoiding any investments in technology or infrastructure

Answer: c. Aligning resource allocation with strategic priorities
Explanation: Ensuring that resources, including finances, are allocated in line with the strategic priorities guarantees that essential projects are funded, promoting sustainability and successful implementation.

355. A key first step in risk management for nurse executives is:
a. Developing risk mitigation strategies.
b. Completing an annual report.
c. Identifying potential risks in clinical and non-clinical areas.
d. Purchasing insurance.

Answer: c. Identifying potential risks in clinical and non-clinical areas.
Explanation: Before risks can be managed, they first need to be identified. Recognizing potential risks is essential to developing tailored strategies for mitigation.

356. When assessing risks, which tool can be valuable in prioritizing them based on their likelihood and potential impact?
a. SWOT Analysis.
b. Risk Matrix.
c. PDSA Cycle.
d. Income Statement.

Answer: b. Risk Matrix.
Explanation: A Risk Matrix is a tool used in risk assessment that ranks risks based on their likelihood of occurrence and potential impact, aiding in prioritizing them.

357. For nurse executives, one of the primary risk mitigation strategies to ensure patient safety is:
a. Investing in the latest medical equipment.
b. Hiring more administrative staff.
c. Regular staff training and competency assessments.
d. Expanding hospital infrastructure.

Answer: c. Regular staff training and competency assessments.
Explanation: Regularly ensuring the clinical competence of nursing staff is paramount to patient safety. Training ensures the staff is equipped with the latest best practices.

358. Which financial document provides a snapshot of an organization's assets, liabilities, and equity at a specific point in time?
a. Income Statement.
b. Cash Flow Statement.
c. Balance Sheet.
d. Risk Matrix.

Answer: c. Balance Sheet.
Explanation: A Balance Sheet shows an organization's financial position at a specific moment, detailing its assets, liabilities, and equity.

359. When forecasting for future financial needs, a nurse executive should consider:
a. Only historical financial data.
b. New clinical initiatives and potential changes in patient volume.
c. Solely the recommendations of external consultants.
d. Financial trends in unrelated industries.

Answer: b. New clinical initiatives and potential changes in patient volume.
Explanation: Accurate forecasting in healthcare requires consideration of future clinical programs, projected changes in patient volume, and other relevant internal factors.

360. Budget variances in a nursing department can result from:
a. Fluctuations in patient census.
b. Changes in government regulations.
c. Inaccurate forecasting of equipment costs.
d. All of the above.

Answer: d. All of the above.
Explanation: Various factors, both internal and external, can impact the actual expenses and revenues compared to budgeted amounts, resulting in variances.

361. In financial management, which statement offers insights into the inflows and outflows of cash over a period?
a. Income Statement.
b. Cash Flow Statement.
c. Balance Sheet.
d. Risk Matrix.

Answer: b. Cash Flow Statement.
Explanation: The Cash Flow Statement provides detailed information about cash inflows and outflows from operations, investments, and financing over a given period.

362. Which strategy can assist nurse executives in managing financial risks related to potential lawsuits?
a. Adopting evidence-based clinical practices.
b. Reducing staff.
c. Increasing marketing spend.
d. Investing in unrelated industries.

Answer: a. Adopting evidence-based clinical practices.
Explanation: Implementing and adhering to evidence-based clinical practices can reduce the risk of adverse patient events and associated legal actions.

363. When reviewing an Income Statement, a nurse executive identifies that revenues have increased, but net income has decreased. This could be due to:
a. Reduced patient volume.
b. Inefficient utilization of resources.
c. An increase in investments.
d. Decrease in liabilities.

Answer: b. Inefficient utilization of resources.
Explanation: If revenues have risen but net income has decreased, it indicates that costs have gone up, potentially due to resource inefficiencies or other added expenses.

364. To effectively manage risks in nursing, regular reviews should be conducted to:
a. Only address financial issues.
b. Identify new risks and assess the effectiveness of current mitigation strategies.
c. Focus solely on patient complaints.
d. Compare with other industries.

Answer: b. Identify new risks and assess the effectiveness of current mitigation strategies.
Explanation: Regular reviews in risk management help identify emerging risks and assess the efficiency of existing risk mitigation tactics, ensuring timely adjustments.

*And there you have it—a whirlwind journey through the vast and intricate landscape of the ANCC Nurse Executive realm. From the ebbs and flows of healthcare economics to the intricate dance of risk management, we've ventured together, deciphering the maze of policies and delving deep into the heart of strategic management.*

*But remember, this guide is just that—a guide. Real mastery comes from the synthesis of knowledge and experience. The true test is the everyday application, where theory meets practice, and where challenges become triumphs.*

*Your dreams are within reach. Those moments of doubt, the days when things don't go as planned, remember that they don't define you. Failures? Consider them stepping stones, not stumbling blocks. Every great nurse executive has faced them and emerged stronger, wiser, and more resilient.*

*As for those fears you might be harboring? It's natural. The path you're on isn't an easy one, but the rewards? Oh, they're monumental. With every policy you shape and every decision you make, you're sculpting the future of healthcare, ensuring that patient care remains at its zenith.*

*Suspicions, too, have their place. They keep you on your toes, urging you to question, to probe deeper, to never settle. But also know when to trust, when to let go, and when to lead with confidence.*

*So, as you stand on this threshold, equipped with knowledge and brimming with passion, know that you're not alone. This journey you're on is shared by many, and by lifting each other up, the sky's the limit.*

*Go forth with a heart full of hope and a mind sharp as a tack. Here's wishing you not just success, but fulfillment, growth, and endless moments of pride and joy. Take the world by storm, dear Nurse Executive. We're rooting for you every step of the way!*

Printed in the USA
CPSIA information can be obtained
at www.ICGtesting.com
LVHW081244200324
774975LV00007B/128